BEYOND CONSENT

BEYOND CONSENT

Seeking Justice in Research

Edited by

Jeffrey P. Kahn, PhD, MPH

Anna C. Mastroianni, JD, MPH

Jeremy Sugarman, MD, MPH, MA

SECOND EDITION

OXFORD
UNIVERSITY PRESS

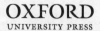

OXFORD
UNIVERSITY PRESS

Oxford University Press is a department of the University of Oxford. It furthers
the University's objective of excellence in research, scholarship, and education
by publishing worldwide. Oxford is a registered trade mark of Oxford University
Press in the UK and certain other countries.

Published in the United States of America by Oxford University Press
198 Madison Avenue, New York, NY 10016, United States of America.

© Oxford University Press 2018

CIP data is on file at the Library of Congress
ISBN 978–0–19–999068–9

9 8 7 6 5 4 3 2 1

Printed by WebCom, Inc., Canada

To our mentor and source of great professional inspiration, Ruth Faden, who brought us together, and who seems to accomplish more than seems realistically possible with humor, grace, wisdom, and humanity.

PREFACE

When we began work on the first edition of *Beyond Consent* in the late 1990s, justice issues arising in research were capturing the attention of the public and policymakers. Patients were making powerful pleas for inclusion in research, Congressional hearings were being held on research with psychiatric patients, debates were focused on the acceptability of conducting research in emergency settings, and new laws and guidances were being implemented to include women and racial and ethnic groups in research. Those controversies and events prompted our work on this book. Some twenty years later, some of those issues have persisted. But different issues have also arisen, prompted by new global health threats, slowed public funding, research scandals, disciplinary actions, research uses of social media, and public advocacy, among other events and circumstances. This second edition seems as relevant as the first.

As we considered how best to approach this edition, we thought it appropriate to invite authors from the first edition to update their chapters with current controversies, to reflect on their earlier predictions, and to look forward into the future once again. In some cases, they brought in other experts as coauthors, with helpful additional perspectives for readers. We also recruited an author to offer a fresh consideration on how to think about concepts and theories of justice in research, and we also added new chapters to address considerations of research involving communities and persons who lack decision-making capacity.

We would be remiss if we did not acknowledge that the foundational approach reflected in this edition emanates from important guidance from—and the influences of—our friends and colleagues Ruth Faden and Madison Powers. We also want to thank Jaclyn Greenberg, Victoria Parker and Shelby Ross at the University of Washington for their expertise and assistance with research and preparation of the manuscript. And lastly, we thank Peter Ohlin, our editor at Oxford University Press, for shepherding this project to completion.

J.P.K.

A.C.M.

J.S.

CONTENTS

List of Contributors   xi

1. Examining Justice in Research: An Introduction and
   Overview
   JEFFREY P. KAHN, ANNA C. MASTROIANNI, AND
   JEREMY SUGARMAN   1

2. The Evolving Story of Justice in Research
   ERIC M. MESLIN AND CHARLES R. McCARTHY   13

3. Justice and Research with the Vulnerable Sick
   BARUCH A. BRODY AND NEAL W. DICKERT   36

4. Justice and Research in Populations with Cognitive
   Impairment
   SCOTT KIM   54

5. Justice and Pediatric Research
   LAINIE FRIEDMAN ROSS AND ROBERT M. NELSON   72

6. Justice and Women's Participation in Research
   NANCY KASS AND ANNE DRAPKIN LYERLY   91

7. Justice, Race, and Racism in Research
   PATRICIA A. KING   112

8. Justice, Research, and Communities
   KATHERINE F. KING AND JAMES V. LAVERY   135

9. Justice and Research with Convenient and Captive
   Populations
   JONATHAN D. MORENO   152

10. Justice and Global Research
    RUTH MACKLIN   169

11. Theorizing Justice in Health Research
    YASHAR SAGHAI   187

12. Pursuing Justice in Research
    JEFFREY P. KAHN, ANNA C. MASTROIANNI, AND
    JEREMY SUGARMAN   208

Index   217

CONTRIBUTORS

Baruch A. Brody, PhD
Andrew Mellon Professor of
   Humanities, Rice University
Emeritus Distinguished Service
   Professor, Baylor College of
   Medicine
Houston, Texas

Neal W. Dickert, MD, PhD
Assistant Professor, Emory
   University School of Medicine
Atlanta, Georgia

Jeffrey P. Kahn, PhD, MPH
Andreas C. Dracopoulos Director,
   Johns Hopkins Berman Institute
   of Bioethics
Baltimore, Maryland

Nancy Kass, ScD
Phoebe R. Berman Professor of
   Bioethics and Public Health,
   Johns Hopkins Berman Institute
   of Bioethics
Baltimore, Maryland

Scott Kim MD, PhD
Senior Investigator, Department
   of Bioethics, National Institutes
   of Health
Bethesda, Maryland

Katherine F. King, PhD
Project Manager, Redstone
   Strategy Group
Boulder, Colorado

Patricia A. King, JD
Carmack Waterhouse Professor of
   Law, Medicine, Ethics, and Public
   Policy, Georgetown University
   Law Center
Washington, DC

James V. Lavery, PhD
Conrad N. Hilton Chair in
   Global Health Ethics, Emory
   University
Atlanta, Georgia

Anne Drapkin Lyerly, MD, MA
Professor of Social Medicine,
   University of North Carolina at
   Chapel Hill
Chapel Hill, North Carolina

Ruth Macklin, PhD
Professor Emerita, Albert Einstein
   College of Medicine
Bronx, New York

Anna C. Mastroianni, JD, MPH
Professor, University of Washington
  School of Law
Seattle, Washington

Charles R. McCarthy, PhD
Richmond, Virginia

Eric M. Meslin, PhD, FCAHS
President and CEO, Council of
  Canadian Academies
Ottawa, Ontario

Jonathan D. Moreno, PhD
David and Lyn Silfen University
  Professor of Ethics, University of
  Pennsylvania
Philadelphia, Pennsylvania

Robert M. Nelson, MD, PhD
Senior Director of Pediatric Drug
  Development, Child Health
  Innovation and Leadership
  Department, Johnson & Johnson
Raritan, New Jersey

Lainie Friedman Ross, MD, PhD
Carolyn and Matthew Bucksbaum
  Professor of Clinical Ethics
  University of Chicago
Chicago, Illinois

Yashar Saghai, MA, PhD
Research Scholar, Johns Hopkins
  Berman Institute of Bioethics
Baltimore, Maryland

Jeremy Sugarman, MD, MPH, MA
Harvey M. Meyerhoff Professor of
  Bioethics and Medicine, Johns
  Hopkins Berman Institute of
  Bioethics
Baltimore, Maryland

1 EXAMINING JUSTICE IN RESEARCH

AN INTRODUCTION AND OVERVIEW

Jeffrey P. Kahn
Anna C. Mastroianni
Jeremy Sugarman

Claims about justice in research abound. Patients with life-threatening, devastating diseases demand access to experimental treatments.[1-6] Advocacy groups' lobbying for funding for research on particular diseases and conditions increasingly play a pivotal role in designing and conducting research.[7,8] Federal research policies require accounting for the gender, race, and ethnicity of those enrolled in research.[9,10] Sponsors and researchers more commonly consider their obligations to research participants and their communities when research concludes.[11,12]

Those claims all point to a series of critical questions related to justice: What does fairness demand in terms of selecting the types of research that are conducted, and with which participant populations? Ethically and practically, which individuals and groups should be included and which excluded? Who should decide, and pursuant to what criteria? How should fairness be interpreted in regards to the distribution of benefits to those participating in research, and to the relevance of that research for society? What are the impacts and implications of both real and perceived injustices in biomedical research on recruiting and retaining research participants? On public perception of research? And, on health care for the population generally? Such questions are both conceptually and practically difficult. Nonetheless, ethically acceptable research is contingent on answers to these questions.

This is not to say that the importance of justice is only recently recognized. Indeed, justice has long been a crucial part of the ethical analyses of research. For instance, in 1979 the National Commission for the Protection of Human Subjects of Biomedical and Behavioral Research specified in the *Belmont Report* the need to consider the principle of justice as well as the principles of respect for persons and beneficence.[13] The National Commission found two senses of justice to be important:

> Who ought to receive the benefits of research and bear its burdens? This is a question of justice in the sense of "fairness in distribution" or "what is deserved." An injustice occurs when some benefit to which a person is entitled is denied without good reason or when some burden is imposed unduly. Another way of conceiving the principle of justice is that equals ought to be treated equally. (p. 23194)[13]

In the context of research, the National Commission invoked the principle of justice in determining the fair selection of subjects. That selection was considered at the individual and societal levels:

> Individual justice in the selection of subjects would require that researchers exhibit fairness: thus they should not offer potentially beneficial research only to some patients who are in their favor or select only "undesirable" persons for risky research. Social justice requires that distinction be drawn between classes of subjects that ought, and ought not, to participate in any particular kind of research, based on the ability of members of that class to bear burdens and on the appropriateness of placing further burdens on already burdened persons. (p. 23196)[13]

Holding that view of justice, the National Commission characterized certain populations ("racial minorities, the economically disadvantaged, the very sick, and the institutionalized") as "vulnerable," thereby requiring special protection (p. 23197).[13] The dominant interpretation of justice used by the National Commission, as well as by many others wrestling with issues related to research with human subjects at that time, emphasized approaches that would protect against potential harms of being included in research.

Although the principle of justice has long been an important part of research ethics, its interpretation and accompanying applications continue to evolve. For example, it is now not uncommon for patients to desire access to experimental interventions and to demand access to research.[2-3,6] Here, justice is viewed as fairness in access rather than protection from risk. As such, there need to be considerations that go well beyond simply obtaining consent to the risks and burdens of that research: they must include creating opportunities for fair access to research and its potential benefits, while simultaneously developing mechanisms of protecting subjects from exploitation. That balancing is a critical challenge for research ethics.

In other instances claims may be made for compensatory justice. For example, a broad claim for compensatory justice might call for additional research efforts directed at understanding the problems faced by groups, or classes of persons that have not had access to research in the past.[14-17] At an individual level, a claim for compensatory justice might relate to developing a means of compensating those who were in some way injured or harmed in the context of research.[18-21] Thus, a comprehensive assessment of research with human subjects necessitates incorporating multiple considerations of justice.

Chapter Previews

The chapters in this volume offer an opportunity for in-depth examination of the concept of justice in research. At times, that requires making implicit aspects of justice more explicit. At other times, it requires examining why a particular approach to justice dominated public discourse and policy development.

Chapter 2 begins the examination, with Eric Meslin and Charles McCarthy sketching a history of the federal policy stance toward justice in research that followed from, among other events, the revelation of scandals in research with human subjects. Punctuating this history is a series of cases that, when brought to public attention, greatly influenced attitudes and approaches toward research. Some of the most notorious cases involve violations of justice in research: African American men in the Tuskegee Syphilis Study from whom treatment was withheld even after effective antibiotic therapies became available; elderly patients in the Jewish Chronic Disease Hospital who were injected with live cancer cells without their consent; and intellectually disabled children in the Willowbrook State School who were deliberately exposed to hepatitis. In such cases research subjects seem to have been selected because of their relative lack of power compared to other potential, and less vulnerable, research subjects. In each of those cases, the risks or burdens of participation were borne by the subjects, yet there was very little prospect of direct benefit to them. Indeed, in light of such cases, it is not surprising that the regulatory stance adopted pursuant to the United States' landmark National Research Act of 1974 was a protectionist one.

On the heels of the *Final Report* of the Tuskegee Syphilis Study Ad Hoc Advisory Panel, the National Commission for the Protection of Human

Subjects invoked two primary notions of justice: fairness in distribution of burdens and benefits, and equals ought to be treated equally.[13] Those notions provided conceptual support for the largely protectionist federal policy toward research. Nearly twenty years later, in response to a variety of forces and influences, research policies began to emphasize inclusion of research subjects—not only in terms of actual participation in research but also in terms of research design—in setting research priorities and making funding decisions. The shift in emphasis toward inclusion of research subjects has focused considerations of justice in somewhat different ways, with effects on not only who is included in research but how research is performed, reviewed, and overseen. Meslin and McCarthy examine those issues through the lenses of distributive, compensatory, and procedural justice, and the various relevant actors for each.

Following that historical overview are a series of chapters, each examining how the concept of justice has been either ignored or applied in the selection of particular groups of research subjects, with suggestions about how the concept should be applied today and in the future. The groups examined include patients, persons with cognitive impairment, children, women, racial groups, captive and convenient groups, communities, and global populations. Of course, those groupings overlap, sometimes substantially, challenging the ability to characterize every relevant consideration of justice for any particular grouping. The text's overall examination does not capture the full range of relevant considerations that must be given to other important populations, such as people with disabilities, the elderly, and LGBT (lesbian, gay, bisexual, and transgendered persons)—groups that have largely eluded special attention regarding inclusion in research, despite their unique concerns. In addition, the claims and uses of the concept of justice vary across the chapters, demonstrating the complexity—and utility—of the concept. This should not be terribly surprising, since such divergent claims have long been part of conceptual work on justice. In the *Nichomachean Ethics*, Aristotle used two definitions for justice: (1) "the whole of virtue" and (2) "fairness in distribution."[22] The remaining chapters in this volume examine and apply each or both definitions in their focus on particular populations.

In Chapter 3, Baruch Brody and Neal Dickert examine questions of justice from the perspective of the vulnerable sick. In this context, they touch on some competing values of justice: the social need for research, potential benefit to subjects, and their protection from exploitation and harm. In actual cases none of those values is controlling on its own. Rather, Brody and Dickert argue that a "balancing" conception of those values, and of the competing claims of protection and access, must be employed.

The authors use the balancing conception in examining three cases, engaging policies that reflect this conception of justice. First, they consider the conduct of research on acute, emergent illnesses, such as heart attacks and strokes, where clinical circumstances may preclude obtaining informed consent. Despite a strong moral obligation to obtain informed consent for research, the competing values of access to experimental treatments that may benefit the subject and the social need to conduct this research must also be considered, and in so doing, highlight the complexities of that context. Second, in describing the push for effective treatments for HIV infection and cancer at times when prognoses are poor, Brody and Dickert demonstrate how the balancing conception of justice accommodates the desperate claims of those patients for whom there is not an established effective treatment with the social need for sound scientific data so that other persons are not exposed to the risk of experimental treatments that have not been adequately tested. Third, Brody and Dickert examine Phase I oncology trials, using the balancing conception of justice to suggest alternative trial designs that may be more commensurate with the concerns of patient-subjects than those that employ traditional designs.

In Chapter 4, Scott Kim examines and analyzes questions about when and under what criteria research participation by individuals with progressive loss of cognitive function could be ethically acceptable, focusing on patients with Alzheimer disease (AD). Kim first examines the history of research involving human subjects with decisional impairment, focusing on the injustices experienced by them, and the longstanding absence of policy directed at the inclusion of decisionally impaired individuals in research. Until relatively recently, those abuses took place in research that was unrelated to participants' primary condition of cognitive impairment. Those injustices are now being addressed by ensuring that those with decisional impairment are excluded from research when the research can instead be performed with participants capable of consent.

Kim notes, however, that there remains an unprecedented need for more research on diseases, ailments, and treatments related to decisional impairment, and therefore a need to create ethically acceptable (including more equitable) approaches for research participation by those with AD and other decisional impairments. He examines the merits and practical considerations of using families and intimates as surrogate decision-makers, followed by important policy recommendations to prevent unjust exclusion of individuals with decisional impairment from research participation.

Chapter 5, authored by Lainie Friedman Ross and Robert Nelson, raises some of the challenging aspects of justice in research involving children. On the one hand, our intuitions may weigh on the side of protection since children are not able to provide meaningful informed consent to participate in research. On the other, such a stance would preclude children from the potential benefit of research, both as individuals and as a group. Just as in the case of emergency research with adults who are not capable of giving consent, at an individual level certain children would be deprived of the possibility of benefiting from new therapies if research is not permitted. Moreover, if research with children is not conducted, children, as a group, will subsequently not have access to safe and effective treatments.

Despite those real concerns, the history of research with children, along with our intuitions that children ought to be protected, suggest a need for a balanced and considered approach. Ross and Nelson begin the chapter with an account of some of the most notorious cases in research ethics involving institutionalized children: the aforementioned Willowbrook study, where subjects were infected with hepatitis, and studies at the Fernald School where subjects were fed radioactive oatmeal. Given cases such as these, it is not surprising that federal regulatory policy historically leaned toward protection, delineating the limited situations in which research with children would be acceptable. Considerable controversy surrounds this approach since other standards may be more responsive to claims about justice that support increased access and greater inclusion of children in research. Other standards might set the level of acceptable risk differently, such as at the level of risks encountered in daily life, the level of risk determined by individual parents to be acceptable, or simply at whatever risk is assented to when a child reaches a specific age. Controversies surrounding the determination of whether it is acceptable to conduct clinical research in a range of pediatric populations, and with a range of therapies or therapeutic approaches, make it clear that understanding those competing methods of determining risk is critical. Even with more recent policy pronouncements promoting the inclusion of children in research, the extent to which children are both given access to, or are protected from, research hinges upon such an assessment of risks.

Chapter 6, authored by Nancy Kass and Anne Drapkin Lyerly, shifts the focus to women. As in the case of children, until relatively recently, many women had not been included in research. One explanation is founded in notions of fetal protection—a presumption that every woman could become pregnant during a research study, potentially subjecting a future child to an otherwise avoidable risk of harm. Such a stance might not seem terribly surprising in the wake of the tragedy of the early 1960s in which women who had received thalidomide outside of the clinical trial context while they were pregnant later gave birth to infants with severe malformations. Other explanations for excluding women from research focus on cultural factors (such as the assumption that male functioning is the "normal"), liability concerns of research sponsors related to potential fetal harm, and a lack of female leadership in science and medicine.

Historical justifications aside, as in the case of children, such an exclusion may affect women as individuals and as part of a group when it comes to their ability to receive safe and effective medical care. Kass and Lyerly use three case examples to demonstrate a range of important considerations regarding justice and women in research. Those examples are derived from research in cardiovascular disease, HIV disease, and pregnancy. In the aggregate, the examples suggest the ongoing need to attend to the appropriate inclusion of women in research. As in the case of the vulnerable sick and with children, this conceptual move from protection to access is mirrored in regulatory and policy statements that should continue to have an influence on the conduct of clinical research.

In parallel with initiatives to include more women in research has been the promulgation of policies to enhance the representation of members of racial and ethnic groups in research. Such is the focus of Chapter 7, authored by Patricia King, which considers issues of race and justice in research, with an emphasis on African Americans. She argues persuasively that implementing justice in that context requires an understanding of African Americans' experiences not only in research but also in society and health care. Her examination of three research cases underscores the pervasiveness of racism present in society—in research practices, institutions, decision-making, and protections. King illuminates the legacy of degrading and exploitative experimentation and research in the African American community, most notably the Tuskegee Syphilis Study but also the saga of the HeLa cell line derived from Henrietta Lacks' cervical cancer and the more recent lead paint study conducted by the Kennedy Krieger Institute in Baltimore. She notes that the African American community's distrust of the research infrastructure is not surprising.

King, who participated in the drafting of the *Belmont Report*,[13] argues for a reexamination of the report's articulation of distributive justice. That ethical calculus hinges on the fair distribution of risk. In that calculus, the need to protect those who are deemed to be vulnerable, in terms of their prior education, socioeconomic status, or relative lack of power, deserves special attention. While concerns about vulnerability are essential, overprotection combined with a lack of trust in the research community may result in a failure to properly address the health needs of those in racial and ethnic groups—clearly another relevant concern about justice. More guidance is needed to attend to inherent power differentials in the researcher-participant relationship and to counter the prevalence of implicit racial bias in research, including the tendency to rely on biological explanations for differences.

Examining issues such as race and racism in research and attending to the important moral claims of those who face other forms of stigma and discrimination make clear the need to consider justice in regards to communities as well as individuals. In Chapter 8, Katherine King and James Lavery review the growing recognition of the roles of communities in research. The power of communities to shape the research enterprise and address concerns related to justice is exemplified by HIV/AIDS activism, which contributed to accelerated pathways for drug approvals and the formal engagement of communities in the research process. On the other hand, the lack of community engagement has contributed to harms in settings such as research with aboriginal populations and genetic research.

King and Lavery present alternative approaches to community engagement, including participatory research, community advisory boards, and direct engagement. As an ethical matter, community engagement serves to extend respect beyond the individual. As a pragmatic matter, those forms of community engagement can help identify risks and benefits that might otherwise be overlooked, thus prompting attention to their mitigation or enhancement, as appropriate, and ultimately furthering research integrity.

In Chapter 9, Jonathan Moreno reflects on the ethical tensions that implicate justice considerations when research includes captive and convenient populations. Prisoners are the paradigmatic example. Prior to the 1970s, prisoners participated in a large number of clinical studies, and were compensated for that participation. Thereafter, when regulatory amendments addressed ethical concerns about exploitation, with particular focus on prisoners' ability to freely consent to participation in a potentially coercive and hierarchical environment, research involving prisoners plummeted. The characteristics of research involving prisoners are relevant for research with other convenient and captive populations as well, including other institutionalized persons, military personnel, and those in status relationships involving power differentials and hierarchical authority, such as students and employees. Decision-making challenges of some institutionalized persons may be further compounded by the condition that prompted their institutionalization, such as profound intellectual disability or debilitating psychiatric illness. Moreno stresses the contribution of historical perspective in his examination of justice in each of those convenient or captive populations. He includes condemnation of recently revealed studies conducted by the United States in Guatemala, which spanned populations that qualify as convenient or captive: prisoners, soldiers, and institutionalized psychiatric patients and Hansen disease patients.

Questions raised by research with convenient and captive populations not only involve distributive justice (i.e., the fair distribution of the burdens and the benefits of research) but also implicate procedural justice, in which the abilities of those to make decisions may be compromised due to their circumstances. While concerns about appropriate protection of such populations are obvious and, to Moreno, rise to the level of a presumption of protectionism, he acknowledges that justice may require research in those populations in limited circumstances to ensure that benefits accrue to them, both to individuals and to the group as a whole. As has been demonstrated in other populations that have been excluded from research studies, without clinical research little will be known about conditions that are unique to these groups.

In Chapter 10, Ruth Macklin delineates some of the vexing justice issues associated with global health research, including the challenges of balancing protection and access, and risks and benefits. The chapter dissects the ethical acceptability of "double standards" in research—whether it is appropriate, for example, for a risk-benefit calculus to vary based on the wealth status of a study site, employing different standards for resource-poor countries versus industrialized countries. Using this lens, Macklin highlights the difficulties inherent in determining whether research is just or unjust. Using three cases, she examines whether there are there circumstances in low- and middle-income countries that are distinctive enough from those in industrialized countries to justify the applications of different ethical standards in research.

The chapter also examines the controversial topic of post-trial responsibilities. When products are ultimately successful, what obligations do sponsors from industrialized countries have to the individuals and communities in which the research was conducted? Perspectives differ, and critics raise competing allegations of paternalism and exploitation. Macklin next focuses on procedural justice considerations, providing examples of when slavish attention to procedural review requirements mandated by the United States may unjustly fail to account for cultural differences internationally.

Armed with those rich descriptions of how justice has been and might be applied in particular populations, in Chapter 11 Yashar Saghai addresses some of the conceptual aspects of justice that seem most relevant to its application in the context of research with human subjects generally. He starts by assessing the usefulness and applicability of principles of justice to examples of research ethics discussed in the other chapters, and highlights aspects he believes will be most salient for more general application. Saghai then lays out the case for a different and complementary approach, which is to examine theories of justice and their applicability to justice issues in health research from both US and global perspectives. He makes the argument that this latter move has the value of applicability to a wider range of topics to be considered within the scope of health research, from basic biomedical sciences to clinical research, public health and health policy, research on health systems, and health-related social and behavioral sciences.

With this conceptual scheme before us, in Chapter 12 we suggest how to pursue and implement justice in the context of research. Such decisions need to be made explicitly at each stage of the research process, ranging from the decisions about research priorities and formulation of research questions, to the design and conduct of research, and the dissemination and use of research findings. Moreover, this effort must involve a wide range of participants in the research enterprise, including researchers, research subjects, IRB members, institutional administrators, policy makers, public and private funders, and pharmaceutical companies. The realization of justice in research will only be achieved through its consideration at every point in the process by all relevant actors.

The chapters in this edition continue, we hope, to advance the discussion of justice in research. Only through such ongoing reflection and related policy action can issues be appropriately addressed, whether they are longstanding and tied to history or newly confronted and resulting from advances in biomedicine, technology, globalization, and other future challenges arising in research.

Notes

1. Wiejer C. Evolving ethical issues in selection of subjects for clinical research. *Cambridge Quarterly of Healthcare Ethics.* 1996;5(3):334–345.
2. Johnson JE. Patient access in research. *Oncology Nursing Forum.* 1982;9(2):81–82.
3. Schuklenk U, Hogan C. Patient access to experimental drugs and AIDS clinical trial designs: ethical issues. *Cambridge Quarterly of Healthcare Ethics.* 1996;5(3):400–409.
4. Kass NE, Taylor HA, King PA. Harms of excluding pregnant women from clinical research: the case of HIV-infected women. *American Journal of Law, Medicine, and Ethics.* 1996;24(1):36–46.
5. Levine C. Women and HIV/AIDS research: the barriers to equity. *IRB: Ethics & Human Research.* 1991;13(1–2):18–22.

6. Darrow JJ, Sarpatwari A, Avorn J, Kesselheim AS. Practical, legal, and ethical issues in expanded access to investigational drugs. *New England Journal of Medicine.* 2015;372:279–286.

7. Genetic Alliance website. http://www.geneticalliance.org/. Accessed December 4, 2017.

8. Patients Like Me website. https://www.patientslikeme.com/. Accessed December 4, 2017.

9. National Institutes of Health. NIH policy and guidelines on the inclusion of women and minorities as subjects in clinical research—amended, October 2001. https://grants.nih.gov/grants/funding/women_min/guidelines_amended_10_ 2001.htm. Accessed December 4, 2017.

10. US Food and Drug Administration. Collection of race and ethnicity data in clinical trials: guidance for industry and Food and Drug Administration staff. http:// www.fda.gov/ucm/groups/fdagov-public/@fdagov-afda-gen/documents/document/ucm126396.pdf. Published October 2016. Accessed December 4, 2017.

11. World Medical Association. Declaration of Helsinki: ethical principles for medical research involving human subjects. *JAMA.* 2013;310(20):2191–2194:Item 34.

12. Cohen ERM, O'Neill JM, Joffres M, Upshur REG, Mills E. Reporting of informed consent, standard of care and post-trial obligations in global randomized intervention trials: a systematic survey of registered trials. *Developing World Bioethics.* 2009;9(2):74–80.

13. National Commission for the Protection of Human Subjects of Biomedical and Behavioral Research. The Belmont Report: Ethical principles and guidelines for the protection of human subjects of research. *Federal Register.* 1979;44(76):23192–23197.

14. Kass NE, Taylor HA, King PA. Harms of excluding pregnant women from clinical research: the case of HIV-infected women. *Journal of Law, Medicine & Ethics.* 1996;24(1):36–46.

15. Levine C. Women and HIV/AIDS research: the barriers to equity. *IRB: Ethics & Human Research.* 1991;13(1/2):18–22.

16. Corbie-Smith G, Moody-Ayers S, Thrasher AD. Closing the circle between minority inclusion in research and health disparities. *Archives of Internal Medicine.* 2004;164(13):1362–1364.

17. Goering S, Holland S, Fryer-Edwards K. Genetic research practices with marginalized communities. *Hastings Center Report.* 2008;38(2):43–53.

18. Mastroianni A, Faden R, Federman D, eds. *Women and Health Research: Ethical and Legal Issues of Including Women in Clinical Studies.* Vol. 1. Washington, DC: National Academy Press; 1994.

19. President's Commission for the Study of Ethical Problems in Medicine and Biomedical and Behavioral Research. *Report.* Washington, DC: US Government Printing Office; 1982. *Compensating for Research Injuries: The Ethical and Legal*

Implications of Programs to Redress Injured Subjects. Vol. 1. https://repository.library.georgetown.edu/handle/10822/559342. Accessed December 4, 2017.

20. Steinbrook R. Compensation for injured research subjects. *New England Journal of Medicine*. 2006;354(18):1871–1873.

21. Henry LM. Moral gridlock: conceptual barriers to no-fault compensation for injured research subjects. *Journal of Law, Medicine & Ethics*. 2013;41(2):411–423.

22. Aristotle. *The Nicomachean Ethics*. Book V. Ross WD, trans-ed. Oxford, England: Oxford University Press; 2009.

2 THE EVOLVING STORY OF JUSTICE IN RESEARCH

Eric M. Meslin
Charles R. McCarthy

The concept of justice has always invoked powerful moral sentiments, particularly when applied to those at risk of exploitation or harm in research. Those sentiments manifest in different ways, such as calls for fair distribution of benefits, just compensation, or impartial procedures for recruitment of research participants. Sometimes, the moral sentiment of justice requires the acknowledgement of and respect for the dignity of persons, groups, or communities who are being treated unfairly or are at risk of such mistreatment. Just as the ideas of justice can be seen in many political movements in the United States (e.g., the civil rights, antiwar, and women's movements), so too can they be seen in US federal research policy for the protection of human subjects. In this chapter we focus on justice by examining its historical role in US federal research policy governing the protection of human subjects in research. As a historical starting point, we first consider the early expressions of concern for the rights and welfare of research participants that followed revelations of unethical research sponsored or conducted by the US government. We show how those justice considerations have persisted over more than four decades through regulations and other policy statements on a range of issues, including fair subject selection, distribution of risk and benefit, compensation for injury, and the procedural mechanisms of the research oversight system itself.

The remainder of this chapter is organized into three sections: first we explain how federal research regulations incorporated the idea of *distributive justice*. The role of justice played here is seen through the requirements of fair selection of human subjects recruited to participate in research, and the distribution of the risks and potential benefits of that research participation. These ideas may seem obvious at the beginning of the twenty-first century, but they were novel when first codified in US federal research policy.

Second, we discuss how justice has played a role in policy to remedy exploitation or unintended harm in research. This is the idea of *compensatory justice* and we describe the efforts to implement a federal policy for compensating human subjects injured in research. We also draw attention to the use of apology as a means to offer a moral remedy to those harmed in research even when no financial or other legal remedy is offered.

Finally, we turn to the role of *procedural justice* in federal policy—namely that fair procedures should be used to determine who should be included (or excluded) from research, and that decision-making structures to approve research should be impartial. US research policy places great emphasis on fair procedures, so it is noteworthy that in important ways these procedures have had to change over time to be responsive to concerns about justice. We discuss the changing emphasis on the inclusion of women and children as an example of this changing view about inclusion in research, and reflect on the use of institutional review boards (IRBs) as impartial expert decision-makers assessing the ethical acceptability of research.

A Historical Examination

The history of research involving human subjects in the United States includes many stories of exceptional scientific progress that led to remarkable interventions, from the polio vaccine to sophisticated surgical techniques. But the history also includes painful cases of unethical and exploitative treatment of human beings who were the subjects of research. Indeed, these stories have become so well-known and documented that they have become part of the story of the origin of the US federal system for the protection of human subjects. Importantly, these were cases that arose in the United States, undertaken by prominent scientists and in several cases sponsored by the federal government, and that occurred years after the horrific cases of experimentation on human beings revealed during the Nuremberg War Crimes Trials.

Among the first set of scandals in the United States to receive public attention post-Nuremberg were twenty-two cases of unethical research documented by Harvard anesthesiologist Henry Beecher in an exposé he published in the 1966 *New England Journal of Medicine (NEJM)*.[1] Beecher described cases in which babies were exposed to risk, consent was not obtained, and where known effective treatments were withheld. Beecher's status as a prominent physician, and the use of the *NEJM* as a vehicle for disseminating these cases contributed to a broader awareness of the need for a better approach to assuring the ethical integrity of medical research. Interestingly, Beecher himself was not supportive of the idea of formal ethics review committees nor confident that "consent in any fully informed sense" was possible (p. 1354).[1] He was more convinced that the best protection against unjust research was the presence of an "intelligent, informed, conscientious, compassionate, and responsible investigator" (p. 1360).[1]

While Beecher's revelations were shocking to the scientific establishment, few cases carried more gravity or had more influence on the development of US policy for the protection of human subjects than the US Public Health Service's "Study of Untreated Syphilis in the Negro Male" (often referred to as the "Tuskegee Syphilis Study") documented in detail in the report by the Tuskegee Syphilis Study Ad Hoc Advisory Panel of the Department of Health, Education, and Welfare (DHEW) in 1973,[2] and later by James Jones in his 1981 book *Bad Blood*.[3] In July 1972 a story was published in the *New York Times* that described an ongoing study begun in 1932 and carried out by researchers in the US Public Health Service in rural Alabama, the purpose of which was to observe the natural progression of untreated, late-stage syphilis in hundreds of African American men. Their syphilis remained untreated even after the discovery of penicillin in 1943, a drug capable of treating the disease and that was soon widely available for that indication. It is estimated that 28 of the men died as a result of nontreatment and a further 100 suffered other debilitating conditions.[3]

Yet as important to the establishment of US federal policy as the revelations of the Tuskegee Syphilis Study were, other cases were part of the story, many of which were documented by Jay Katz, Alex Capron, and Eleanor Swift Glass in *Experimentation with Human Beings: The Authority of the Investigator, Subject, Profession, and State in the Human Experimentation Process*.[4] Published in 1972, this book remains one of the most comprehensive collections of case studies in medical research and treatment including two of which have become both classics and infamous:

• A study to investigate the effect of the body's immune system when directly exposed to cancer conducted at Brooklyn's Jewish Chronic Disease Hospital in the early 1960s. Immunologist Chester Southam developed a protocol in which elderly, debilitated patients would have live cancer cells injected into their arms to assess the body's response. The patients were not informed that they were being injected with live cancer cells.[4]

• The Willowbrook State School experiments, a series of studies undertaken at what was a residential school in Staten Island, New York, by respected virologist Saul Krugman in which developmentally disabled children were intentionally exposed to hepatitis, some being fed live hepatitis virus and others injected. The Willowbrook experiments were halted in the mid-1960s, but the story of overcrowding, unsanitary conditions, mistreatment of children, and the choice of research population shocked the country when it was the subject of a documentary in 1972 by Geraldo Rivera, at the time a young investigative reporter for WABC-TV in New York.[4]

Like Beecher's *NEJM* article, the Katz, Capron, and Glass 1972 compendium of cases provides important reference points for the development of the federal system for protecting human subjects. In each of these cases, and others, the role justice played was self-evident: people were exploited due to their institutionalized status and limited ability to consent, their rights were violated, and there was little or no recourse to remedy the harms they suffered.

Distributive Justice: From Subject Selection to Benefit Sharing

Considerations of justice can be found in the first published policy regarding research issued in 1953, which pertained to the rights and welfare of normal volunteers who participated in research at the newly opened Clinical Center of the National Institutes of Health (NIH) in Bethesda, Maryland.[5] It is well worth remembering the context for this policy. NIH Director Dr. James Shannon was committed to protecting the rights and welfare of human subjects both because he placed high value on the rights of research subjects, and because he understood that failure to protect them could lessen or undermine congressional support for the fight against disease waged by the NIH. He said, "[Research] departs from the conventional physician-patient relationship . . . the patient's good has been substituted for by the need to develop new knowledge. . . ." (p. 30).[6] On February 8, 1965, Surgeon General William Stewart issued *PHS Policy and Procedure Order # 129*. The PHS policy was amended several times until finally in 1971 it was expanded and extended to cover all research conducted or supported by the DHEW.[7]

The PHS policy and the *Final Report* of the Tuskegee Syphilis Study Ad Hoc Advisory Panel captured public and congressional attention. Newly elected Senator Edward (Ted) Kennedy (D-MA) held a series of hearings over a period of more than three years that examined many of the scandals previously reported as well as proposals for preventing them in the future. Following these hearings Congress passed the *National Research Act*[8] on July 12, 1974, which, among other things, established a national commission and authorized it to:

- conduct a comprehensive investigation and study to identify the basic ethical principles which should underlie the conduct of biomedical and behavioral research involving human subjects; and
- develop guidelines which should be followed in such research to assure that it is conducted in accordance with such principles.

The US National Commission for the Protection of Human Subjects of Biomedical and Behavioral Research (National Commission) in its 1979 *Belmont Report*[9] subsequently articulated a distributive formulation of justice explained as follows:

> Who ought to receive the benefits and burdens of research and bear its burdens? This is a question of justice, in the sense of "fairness in distribution" or "what is deserved." An injustice occurs when some benefit to which a person is entitled is denied without good reason or when some burden is imposed unduly. Another way of conceiving the principle of justice is that equals ought to be treated equally. (p. 23194)[9]

While this chapter updates the role of justice in the history of federal research policy, we defer to later chapters for some of the more detailed assessments of justice in regard to particular populations. However, the *Belmont Report* provides a concrete locus for the explicit discussion of two aspects of justice. First, the importance of scrutinizing the selection of research participants recruited to participate in studies in order to determine whether some groups (e.g., welfare patients, particular racial and ethnic groups, or persons confined to institutions) are being selected simply because of their easy availability, their compromised situation, or the ability to exploit or manipulate them, rather than for reasons related to their suitability as research subjects for the question being studied. Second, whenever research is supported by public funds, justice demands both that no one group be disproportionately burdened by the risks of research or be recruited into research whose potentially beneficial research findings will not apply to them.

While the term "justice" does not appear in US federal research regulations, the explanation in the *Belmont Report* of how justice is applied can be found throughout federal research policy. For example, the regulation describing "Criteria for IRB Approval of Research" (§46.111(a)(3))[10] to date remains unchanged since it was first introduced in 1981 and includes this provision:

Selection of subjects is equitable. In making this assessment the IRB should take into account the purposes of the research and the setting in which the research will be conducted and should be particularly cognizant of the special problems of research involving vulnerable populations, such as children, prisoners, pregnant women, mentally disabled persons, or economically or educationally disadvantaged persons.

These criteria for IRB review also find specific application in the additional regulatory protections applying to Pregnant Women, Neonates and Fetuses ("Subpart B"); Prisoners ("Subpart C"); and Children ("Subpart D").[10] The protections applicable to each of these populations emphasize the ethical obligations consistent with the *Belmont Report*'s principle of justice, including not to exploit research participants, nor to target them for involvement in research because they are easier to recruit, more administratively accessible, or less likely to decline. An explicit version of this regulatory requirement is found in protections related to prisoners, "Additional duties of the Institutional Review Boards where prisoners are involved," where IRBs are instructed that:

Procedures for the selection of subjects within the prison are fair to all prisoners and immune from arbitrary intervention by prison authorities or prisoners. (§46.305(a)(4))[10]

Novel as it was at that time for a federal policy commission created by Congress to define and apply a complex philosophical principle, the National Commission's attention to justice is now seen as incomplete in important ways. As Patricia King has explained, the National Commission's focus on justice included only those issues arising from subject selection in studies, and "ignored other aspects of justice, notably compensatory justice, that arguably were relevant to its task of protecting human subjects" (p. 137).[11] We will turn to compensatory justice below but note that the *Belmont Report* did not anticipate two other issues: the first is the opportunity to distribute benefits to individuals arising from the study *after* it is completed; the second is the importance of sharing research data among scientists.

Access to Benefits Following a Study

By the mid-1990s the ethics of international research attracted increased scholarly and policy attention stimulated in part by a study conducted in the US by the AIDS Clinical Trials Group. The study, ACTG 076, showed a marked decrease in the risk of mother-to-child transmission of HIV and was recommended to become the accepted standard of care. However, questions arose about whether this standard should or could be implemented in low and middle income countries (LMICs).[12,13] The ensuing controversy about the design of new studies regarding mother-to-child transmission of HIV in LMICs is discussed in greater detail elsewhere in this volume (see Chapter 10), but the ACTG 076 case and subsequent discussions related to it also highlighted the need to take a broader view of the ethical obligations related to research. While there was prior acknowledgment of ethical obligations that apply during research (e.g., ensuring equitable selection of participants, minimizing risk, and obtaining voluntary consent), there was emerging recognition in academic and regulatory circles about obligations to participants after a study is completed. For instance, this included deliberation about the obligation to ensure that research participants (and their communities) are able to access a medicine shown to be effective in a study. This obligation and the reciprocal right to access benefits—grounded in a principle of justice as reciprocity – has now been reflected in policies and guidelines.

Among the first to take a position on this was President Clinton's National Bioethics Advisory Commission (NBAC), which argued that there was an obligation, grounded in the principle of justice, for the issue of post-trial access to beneficial treatment to be addressed in the design of studies. NBAC recommended:

> Researchers and sponsors in clinical trials should make reasonable, good faith efforts before the initiation of a trial to secure, at its conclusion, continued access for all participants to needed experimental interventions that have been proven effective for the participants. Although the details of the arrangements will depend on a number of factors (including but not limited to the results of a trial), research protocols should typically describe the duration, extent, and financing of such continued access. When no arrangements have been negotiated, the researcher should justify to the ethics review committee why this is the case. (Recommendation 4.1, p. 74)[14]

The recommendation was based on an application of the principle of justice as "reciprocity" articulated as "[w]hat people deserve as a function of what they have contributed to an enterprise or to society" (p. 59):[14]

> In the context of clinical trials, justice as reciprocity could mean that something is owed to research participants even after their participation in a trial has ended, because it is the only through their acceptance of risk and inconvenience that researchers are able to generate findings necessary to advance knowledge and develop new medical interventions. (p. 59)[14]

Others have also weighed in on this issue.[15,16] The Nuffield Council on Bioethics in the UK adopted reasoning similar to NBAC.[17] So too did the

World Medical Association in its 2000 version[18] of the *Declaration of Helsinki* and in subsequent amendments including the most recent 2013 version.[19] No such requirement to consider post-trial obligations to trial participants exists in US regulations.[20]

Data Sharing

Data sharing has been the source of ethical and legal commentary for decades and is widely seen as desirable ethical behavior with demonstrable benefits to science.[21,22] The expectation that data generated in publicly funded studies will be shared has increasingly been codified in policies of international funding agencies.[23] There has been a resurgence of interest in data sharing following the completion of the sequencing of the human genome and the rise of various technologies to use sequence data.[24] In addition, funding agencies have promoted policies of required sharing of data as a condition of obtaining a grant award.[25]

As an example, genomic data sharing, unlike access to experimental medicines, selection of subjects, or distribution of research benefits, has provided a new set of considerations about fairness in the conduct of research that will continue to provoke discussion. Several key policy statements have been adopted for encouraging data sharing by international groups and consortia specifically for genomic data; these include policies adopted in Bermuda (1997),[26] Fort Lauderdale (2003),[27] and Toronto (2009).[28] On August 26, 2014, the NIH released its Final Genomic Data Sharing Policy that "supports the NIH mission and is essential to facilitate the translation of research results into knowledge, products, and procedures that improve human health" (p. 1).[29] While not phrased explicitly in the language of justice, this policy is illustrative of the family of policies that arose from the human genome project that, at their core, were responding to the ethical, legal, and social implications of new genetic technologies.

Compensatory Justice: Remedies for Injury and Apologies for Wrong

At its core, the federal system governing research involving human subjects attempts to strike a balance between two laudable goals: to support the advance of science in the interest of society, and to ensure that individuals who contribute to this effort are treated with the respect to which they are entitled. This is achieved by obtaining informed consent and, as we discuss below, through independent prior ethical review. The attention to justice in US research policy works to assure the fair inclusion of people participating in research. Considerably less policy emphasis is placed on efforts to seek justice afterwards, where efforts are left to the legal system such as pursuing litigation for injury. In the prior section we mentioned one example of this: the ongoing conversation about providing post-trial benefits to participants as a matter of reciprocity for their contribution. But a much older idea has been the subject of conversation for decades: the responsibility for compensating research subjects for harms they have experienced as a result of their participation in research.

Federal policy is mostly silent on this issue. Of the eight basic elements of informed consent required in the federal regulations, two focus on compensation for injury, yet they merely indicate administrative responsibility and do not refer to any formal program of compensation:

> For research involving more than minimal risk, an explanation as to whether any compensation and an explanation as to whether any medical treatments are available if injury occurs and, if so, what they consist of, or where further information may be obtained; . . . An explanation of whom to contact for answers to pertinent questions about the research and research subjects' rights, and whom to contact in the event of a research-related injury to the subject. (§46.116(a)(6),(7))[10]

Current regulations also prohibit exculpatory language in the informed consent process; that is, language that makes the participant "waive or appear to waive any . . . legal rights, or releases or appears to release the investigator, the sponsor, the institution or its agents from liability for negligence" (§46.116).[10]

From early reported examples of abusive or exploitative research involving human subjects that led to the development of the regulatory system itself to more recent exposés, attention to the plight of those injured in research has occupied US research policy discussion for decades.[30] Even the Tuskegee Syphilis Study Ad Hoc Advisory Panel, whose report played an important role in the establishment of the federal system, observed that:

> No policy for the compensation of research subjects harmed as a consequence of their participation in research has been formulated, despite the fact that no matter how careful investigators may be, unavoidable injury to a few is the price society must pay for the privilege of engaging in research which ultimately benefits the many. Remitting injured subjects to the uncertainties of the law court is not a solution. (p. 23)[2]

In the following decades several bioethics commissions, including the President's Commission for the Study of Ethical Problems in Medicine and Biomedical and Behavioral Research (1978–1983),[31] the Advisory Committee on

Human Radiation Experiments (1994–1995),[32] the National Bioethics Advisory Commission (1996–2001),[33] and the Presidential Commission for the Study of Bioethical Issues (2008–2017),[34] each came to similar conclusions: namely, that there is an ethical justification for the federal government to compensate those individuals who, through no fault of their own, are harmed by their voluntary participation in federally sponsored research. Some of these committees made comprehensive recommendations to adopt a no-fault insurance scheme; others recommended further pilot/feasibility studies.[31,33] Meanwhile, scholars continue to provide justifications and policy argumentation,[35] and yet no policy for providing compensatory justice in research has been forthcoming. The National Vaccine Injury Compensation Program was established by the Health Services Research Administration in 1988,[36] but it focused on injury resulting from the provision of preventive health care, not research. That said, as we describe below, while no formal policy exists, there have been instances in which the federal government has compensated persons injured in research.

Apology for Wrongs

Compensation for injury is typically seen in terms of monetary payment and therefore is the most tangible expression of compensatory justice. But for impact, an apology is a formidable action in its own right, especially when uttered by groups or persons in authority. An important example is the first of the Advisory Committee on Human Radiation Experiments' eighteen recommendations following from its investigation of US–sponsored radiation experiments:

> The Advisory Committee recommends . . . that the government deliver a personal, individualized apology and provide financial compensation to subjects (or their next of kin) of human radiation experiments in which efforts were made by the government to keep information secret from these individuals or their families, or from the public, for the purpose of avoiding embarrassment or potential legal liability, or both, and where this secrecy had the effect of denying individuals the opportunity to pursue potential grievances. (p. 512)[32]

Upon receiving the Advisory Committee's report, President Clinton offered an apology:

> The United States of America offers a sincere apology to those of our citizens who were subjected to these experiments, to their families and to their communities. When the government does wrong, we have a moral responsibility to admit it. (p. 1531)[37]

Clinton's apology was coupled with the US government's agreement to pay $4.8 million to twelve victims who were injected with uranium or plutonium in experiments conducted between 1945 and 1947.[38] It was, in the words of then–Secretary of Energy Hazel O'Leary, an effort "to make those who were wronged and harmed whole."[39] Others have described this type of action as *restorative justice*.[40,41] President Clinton's apology for the radiation experiments was not the only time he would use his stature and office to right a wrong for research sponsored by the US government. Nineteen months after the event accepting the Advisory Committee's report at the White House, on Friday, May 16, 1997, Clinton appeared again in the East Room of the White House to express his regrets for the Tuskegee Syphilis Study[42] where he said:

> To the survivors, to the wives and family members, the children and the grandchildren, I say what you know: No power on Earth can give you back the lives lost, the pain suffered, the years of internal torment and anguish. What was done cannot be undone. But we can end the silence. We can stop turning our heads away. We can look at you in the eye and finally say on behalf of the American people, what the United States government did was shameful, and I am sorry. (p. 608)[42]

Clinton's words that day were profound and comprehensive. In addition to his apology offered to the seven remaining survivors and family members, the president apologized "to Macon County, to Tuskegee, to the doctors who have been wrongly associated with the events there . . . [and] to our African American citizens" (p. 608).[42] And just as the apology for the radiation experiments was intended to acknowledge a wrong committed years prior, the Tuskegee Syphilis Study apology acknowledged the wrongs caused by the US government and by the country. While compensation had been provided to many of the victims in a 1974 out-of-court settlement,[43] he also directed that money be set aside for a memorial, and for a bioethics center at Tuskegee University that functions today as the National Center for Bioethics in Research and Health Care.

A final illustration of apology as a form of compensatory justice occurred on October 1, 2010, when US Secretary of State Hillary Clinton and Secretary of Health and Human Services Kathleen Sibelius issued the following statement:

> Although these events occurred more than 64 years ago, we are outraged that such reprehensible research could have occurred under the guise of public health. We deeply regret that it happened, and we apologize to all the individuals who were affected by such abhorrent research practices.[44]

Secretaries Clinton and Sibelius were referring to the revelation that more than sixty years earlier the US government had supported studies conducted by US researchers in Guatemala in which prisoners, prostitutes, children, members of the military, and patients in mental health hospitals were intentionally exposed to different sexually transmitted infections. The revelations had been identified by respected medical historian Susan Reverby in work presented at national meetings and in print.[45] The government's response did not end with the statement by Secretaries Clinton and Sibelius or the personal apology delivered from President Barack Obama to his Guatemalan counterpart President Alvaro Colom, later that same day by telephone. The president also requested his Presidential Commission for the Study of Bioethical Issues to "oversee a thorough fact-finding investigation into the specifics of the US Public Health Service Sexually Transmitted Disease Inoculation Study."[46] The commission's main conclusion makes reference to how its work should be viewed as responsive when confronted with a revelation of a historical injustice:

> The Commission has concluded that the Guatemala experiments involved gross violations of ethics as judged against both the standards of today and the researchers' own understanding of applicable contemporaneous practices. It is the Commission's firm belief that many of the actions undertaken in Guatemala were especially egregious moral wrongs because many of the individuals involved held positions of public institutional responsibility. The best thing we can do as a country when faced with a dark chapter is to bring it to light. (p. v)[47]

Procedural Justice: IRBs, Assurances, and Inclusion of "Vulnerable Subjects"

The third way in which justice has played a role in US research policy is through the procedures embedded in the regulatory structure itself. Two procedures are noteworthy, as they have been embedded in the federal regulations since their inception four decades ago. The first is the use of IRBs as arbiters of the ethical acceptability of research involving human subjects. The second is the application of a recruitment criterion used by IRBs to determine whether research participants have been selected fairly.

Institutional Review Boards

We have noted the important, early role that NIH Director James Shannon played to develop the 1966 PHS policy for the protection of human subjects (often referred to as the "Yellow Book"). Shannon understood that congressional support for biomedical research could end quickly if federally funded research was judged to be unethical and research subjects were seriously injured. Many others on the NIH staff believed that sound scientific method required research investigators to be free "from control, direction, regimentation, and outside interference" (p. 559).[48] Shannon was deeply committed to developing a fair system of support for research involving human subjects and believed that the ". . . absence of written guidelines on the use of investigative drugs or procedures was no longer tolerable . . . " (p. 157).[6] Robert Q. Marston succeeded Shannon as NIH Director. In an address delivered at the University of Virginia, Marston called for sweeping reforms aimed at protecting the rights of the subjects involved in studies, and created a Task Force of Public Health Service Employees to provide protections for vulnerable populations.[49]

Powerful statements like these by NIH leadership provided some of the fuel necessary to energize ongoing public and political discussion about the need to establish a mechanism for preventing research abuses and to assure the protection of the rights and welfare of human subjects in research. Federal regulations protecting human subjects became effective on May 30, 1974, when the Department of Health, Education, and Welfare (DHEW) gave regulatory status to NIH's Yellow Book. It was through these regulations that IRBs were established as a key mechanism to protect the rights and welfare of human subjects in research.

An underappreciated outcome of the National Commission was a recommendation that DHEW take administrative action to require that the guidelines arising from the *Belmont Report* apply to research conducted or supported by DHEW. DHEW accepted the recommendation and codified this expectation in the "Basic Policy," which became final on January 16, 1981, and was periodically revised over the next decade. The "Basic Policy" is codified in regulations promulgated by each federal agency that conducts or supports research, and since 1991 is referred to as the "Common Rule."[10]

Procedural justice figures in the Common Rule by requiring IRBs to include "diversity of the members, including consideration of race, gender, and cultural backgrounds" and to use "[e]very non-discriminatory effort to ensure that no IRB consists entirely of men or entirely of women members of one gender or profession" (§46.107(b)).[10] In this way the federal regulations sought to ensure that there was fair representation on IRBs tasked with assuring human subjects protection. That said, from their inception IRBs have been subjected to scrutiny about whether they reflect principles of democratic representation or are merely professional structures that support institutional goals.[50]

A second way in which procedural justice is reflected in federal policy is through a contractual arrangement called a Federalwide Assurance (FWA) in which institutions agree to comply with all applicable regulations for the protection of human subjects, including the principles in the *Belmont Report*, in return for eligibility to compete for funding of research projects by US federal agencies. The role of justice is obvious: the federal government can place fair conditions on institutions in exchange for their receiving federal research support. Most institutions extend the FWA provisions to all research involving human subjects, irrespective of the funding source. It is noteworthy that from 1995–2000 more than forty institutions received warnings from the federal Office for Protection from Research Risks (OPRR), and a number of prominent institutions lost the privilege to initiate any research involving human subjects.[33]

Inclusion of "Vulnerable" Subjects

Central to the ethical underpinning of the federal research regulations is the recognition that those believed to be at risk of exploitation or harm but who could not protect their own interests were considered "vulnerable" and therefore deserving of additional special protections. This approach might best be described as benevolently paternalistic, based on the idea that those who could not protect themselves needed someone else to protect them. For those unable to consent on their own behalf this made sense, and hence special protections for children were included as a category since they lack the same autonomous decision-making capacity of adults.

But this protectionist approach was also applied to a cluster of others: pregnant women, fetuses, neonates, and prisoners, for reasons discussed elsewhere in this book. Pregnant women were considered vulnerable because of the risks that they would be assuming on behalf of a potential fetus. It is especially noteworthy that those vulnerability concerns were, in practice, extended more broadly to women as a group. All women were in effect treated as potentially pregnant and therefore potentially vulnerable. This approach, however benevolent, may have had an opposite and unjust consequence: it effectively limited research on women's health issues.[51] In 1993, Congress addressed this issue in recognizing that requirements for additional protections for women and children amounted to a type of reverse discrimination and was therefore unjustly denying these groups the possibility of both participating in research and benefiting from it. They also recognized that similar issues applied to racial and ethnic minorities. Congress addressed two of these injustices in the 1993 NIH Revitalization Act where a specific amendment included the following language:

SEC. 492B. (a) Requirement of Inclusion —

(1) In general —In conducting or supporting clinical research for purposes of this title, the Director of NIH shall, subject to subsection (b), ensure that—(A) women are included as subjects in each project of such research; and (B) members of minority groups are included as subjects in such research.[52]

Rather than excluding women and minorities from research, Congress required that they be included in studies unless there were good reasons to exclude them. By 1994, reports from the General Accounting Office (GAO—an investigative arm of the US Congress, now called the Government Accountability Office)[53] and the US Institute of Medicine (IOM—now called the National Academy of Medicine, part of the nongovernmental National Academies of Sciences, Engineering, and Medicine)[54] lent further credence to this change in regulatory philosophy. The GAO found that women were underrepresented in clinical trials and that data from studies involving men were applied to women ignoring physiological differences between men and women that might affect everything from drug dosing to physiology. In response, both the NIH and Food and Drug Administration (FDA) created offices whose missions were to (1) protect and advance the health of women through policy, science, and outreach, and (2) advocate for inclusion of women in clinical trials and analysis of gender/sex effects. Among other benefits, this contributed to a marked increase in the number of studies, including those to address hypertension, anthrax prevention, depression, and infection, during pregnancy.[55]

In March 1998, the NIH further emphasized its commitment to redressing the injustice of effectively excluding children from research when it issued its Policy and Guidelines on the Inclusion of Children as Participants in Research Involving Human Subjects.[56] Several years later, in October 2001, an updated NIH Policy and Guidelines on the Inclusion of Women and Minorities as Subjects in Clinical Research[57] was released, describing the conditions under which vulnerable persons should be included in studies. Importantly, this policy placed procedural justice front and center by requiring that a justification must be provided to an IRB if women and minorities were *not* to be included in research. In particular, the policy opened a door for women to participate in research that had previously been shut by overly protective (if well-intended) regulations. This topic remains an important focus of concern, given that despite major changes in federal regulations and policy there are gaps in research and its application to women's health research, including research addressing the health needs of pregnant women[58] (see Chapter 6).

Federal Advisory Committees

No evolving story of justice in US federal regulations would be complete without describing the role played by federal bioethics advisory committees. Indeed, one of the more innovative experiments in domestic US bioethics policy development can be seen in the use of public committees and commissions to develop, adopt, and apply ethical principles and theories to inform public policy in the health sciences.[59] These commissions used or considered concepts of justice in their deliberations, although we mention only a few here. It is significant that while the National Commission was the first federal bioethics body to define and apply the principle of justice in research, subsequent committees adopted diverse stances on the topic. For example, as Alexander Capron notes in his reflection on the relevance of the *Belmont Report* to the deliberations of the President's Commission for the Study of Ethical Problems in Medicine and Biomedical and Behavioral Research (The President's Commission): "the curious aspect of the *Belmont Report* is that it played virtually no part in the deliberations or conclusions of the President's Commission" (p. 29).[60] Capron, who was the President's Commission's executive director, gave three explanations for the absence of *Belmont*'s principles in their deliberations: (1) the National Commission focused on research, whereas the main emphasis of the President's Commission was on ethical and policy issues in health care; (2) the principles themselves were not seen as useful by commission staff; and (3) the methods used by the President's Commission were less principle-based than they were "highly contextual" (p. 30).[60] However, at least three of this commission's reports focus on topics that included considerations of justice in research: *Protecting Human Subjects*,[61] *Whistleblowing in Biomedical Research*,[62] and *Compensating for Research Injuries*.[31]

In contrast with the President's Commission's curious nonuse of the principle of justice, the 1994–1995 Advisory Committee on Human Radiation Experiments (ACHRE) adopted the *Belmont* principle of justice as one of the "basic ethical principles that are widely accepted and generally regarded as so fundamental as to be applicable to the past as well as the future" (p. 43),[32] and used it as an instrument of policy analysis and research. Of the six principles applied in ACHRE's analysis and policy recommendations, the fifth stated that "one ought to treat people fairly and with equal respect," a formulation broader than the straightforward distributive sense of justice found in the *Belmont Report* (p. 51).[63] The National Bioethics Advisory Commission (NBAC, 1996–2001) contributed in ways both similar to and different from the President's Commission and ACHRE. For example, the idea of revisiting the *Belmont* principles (and proposing to supplement them with an additional principle) was first proposed by then-commissioner Ezekiel Emanuel.[64] While such action was never taken, the *Belmont* principles might be said to have informed NBAC's work but did not determine it. Several of NBAC's reports focused on topics that implicated justice, including *Research Involving Persons with Mental Disorders that May Affect Decisionmaking Capacity* where it recommended that: "An IRB should not approve research protocols targeting persons with mental disorders as subjects when such research can be done with other subjects" (Recommendation 3).[65] When read alongside its justification, there is little doubt that the *Belmont* principle of justice was of greatest concern:

> First it is important, on the grounds of justice and fairness, to discourage any tendency to engage these persons in research simply because they are in some sense more available than others. Second, this prohibition would further reinforce the importance of informed consent in human subjects research. The principles of justice and respect for persons jointly imply that IRBs should not approve research protocols. (Chapter 5)[65]

Conclusion

This chapter discusses the historical role of justice in US research policy by describing three different types of justice—distributive, compensatory, and procedural—by illustrating their influence on different domains of policy related to research on human subjects. In each instance we noted the extent to which justice considerations were visible and prominent, though sometimes more subtle. Taking as a historical starting point the early expressions of concern for the rights and welfare of research participants by key leaders at the NIH and in the US Congress, and then tracing developments following the National Commission's *Belmont Report,* we showed how justice considerations have persisted over more than three decades through policies to ensure fair subject selection, equitable distribution of risk and benefit, compensation for injury, and as procedural mechanisms through the Federalwide Assurance policy and the IRB system itself.

But descriptions of the instruments of justice in policy are not the same as ensuring that justice is being done. Examples abound of important ways in which justice can be effected in federal policy, but remain elusive—like the ongoing calls for a federal policy to compensate those injured in research, or the growing appreciation of an obligation to provide some form of benefit to participants at the end of a clinical trial. We expect that more policy attention will focus on procedural aspects of justice in the coming years because procedures can be modified, agreed to, commented on, implemented, and evaluated. Welcome though these changes will be, assessing whether justice is actually done will be much more difficult.

Notes

1. Beecher HK. Ethics and clinical research. *New England Journal of Medicine.* 1966;274(24):1354–1360.
2. Tuskegee Syphilis Study Ad Hoc Advisory Panel. *Final Report.* Washington, DC: US Department of Health, Education and Welfare; 1973. http://biotech. law.lsu.edu/cphl/history/reports/tuskegee/tuskegee.htm. Accessed December 9, 2017.
3. Jones J. *Bad Blood: The Tuskegee Syphilis Experiment.* New York, NY: Free Press; 1981.
4. Katz J, Capron AM, Glass ES. *Experimentation with Human Beings: The Authority of the Investigator, Subject, Professions, and State in the Human Experimentation Process.* New York, NY: Russell Sage Foundation; 1972.
5. McCarthy CR. The evolving story of justice in federal research policy. In: Kahn JP, Mastroianni AC, Sugarman J, eds. *Beyond Consent: Seeking Justice in Research.* New York, NY: Oxford University Press; 1998:11–31.
6. National Advisory Health Council September 28, 1965 meeting [transcript]. Quoted by: Frankel MS. *Public Policymaking for Biomedical Research: The Case of Human Experimentation* [dissertation]. Washington, DC: George Washington University; 1976.
7. US Department of Health, Education, and Welfare. *The Institutional Guide to DHEW Policy on Protection of Human Subjects.* Washington, DC: US Government Printing Office; 1971. https://archive.org/details/institutionalgui00nati. Accessed December 9, 2017.
8. National Research Act of 1974. Pub L No 93–348, 88 Stat 342.
9. National Commission for the Protection of Human Subjects of Biomedical and Behavioral Research. The Belmont Report: Ethical principles and guidelines for the protection of human subjects of research. *Federal Register.* 1979;44(76):23192–23197.

10. U.S. Department of Health and Human Services. Protection of human subjects. 45 CFR §46. http://www.hhs.gov/ohrp/regulations-and-policy/regulations/45-cfr-46/#. Revised January 15, 2009. Effective July 14, 2009. Accessed December 9, 2017.

11. King PA. Justice beyond *Belmont*. In: Childress JF, Meslin EM, Shapiro HT, eds. *Belmont Revisited: Ethical Principles for Research with Human Subjects*. Washington, DC: Georgetown University Press; 2005:136–147.

12. Lurie P, Wolfe SM. Unethical trials of interventions to reduce perinatal transmission of the human immunodeficiency virus in developing countries. *New England Journal of Medicine*. 1997;337(12):853–856.

13. Varmus H, Satcher D. Ethical complexities of conducting research in developing countries. *New England Journal of Medicine*. 1997;337(14):1003–1005.

14. National Bioethics Advisory Commission. *Ethical and Policy Issues in International Research: Clinical Trials in Developing Countries*. Vol 1. https://bioethicsarchive.georgetown.edu/nbac/clinical/Vol1.pdf. Bethesda, MD: National Bioethics Advisory Commission; 2001. Accessed December 9, 2017.

15. Glantz LH, Annas GJ, Grodin MA, Mariner WK. Research in developing countries: taking "benefit" seriously. *Hastings Center Report*. 1998;28(6):38–42.

16. El Setouhy M, Agbenyega T, Anto F, et al. Moral standards for research in developing countries: from "reasonable availability" to "fair benefits." *Hastings Center Report*. 2004;34(3):17–27.

17. Nuffield Council on Bioethics. *The Ethics of Research Related to Healthcare in Developing Countries*. London, England: Nuffield Council on Bioethics; 2002. http://nuffieldbioethics.org/wp-content/uploads/2014/07/Ethics-of-research-related-to-healthcare-in-developing-countries-I.pdf. Accessed December 9, 2017.

18. World Medical Association. Declaration of Helsinki: ethical principles for medical research involving human subjects. Version 2000. http://www.who.int/bulletin/archives/79(4)373.pdf. Accessed December 9, 2017.

19. World Medical Association. Declaration of Helsinki: ethical principles for medical research involving human subjects. *JAMA*. 2013;310(20):2191–2194.

20. US Department of Health and Human Services. Federal Policy for the Protection of Human Subjects; Final Rule. *Federal Register*. 2017;82(12): 7149–7274.

21. Feinberg SE, Martin ME, Straf ML, eds. *Sharing Research Data*. Washington, DC: National Academy Press; 1985.

22. Benkler Y, Nissenbaum H. Commons-based peer production and virtue. *Journal of Political Philosophy*. 2006;14(4):394–419.

23. Kaye J, Heeney C, Hawkins N, de Vries J, Boddington P. Data sharing in genomics—reshaping scientific practice. *Nature Review Genetics*. 2009;10: 331–335.

24. Kaye J, Boddington P, de Vries J, et al. *Ethical, Legal and Social Issues Arising from the Use of GWAS in Medical Research*. Oxford, England: University of Oxford;

2009. https://wellcome.ac.uk/sites/default/files/wtx058032.pdf. Accessed December 9, 2017.

25. Tenopir C, Allard S, Douglass K, et al. Data sharing by scientists: practices and perceptions. *PLoS ONE*. 2011;6(6):e21101.

26. Wellcome Trust. Summary of the report of the second international strategy meeting on human genome sequencing, Bermuda, 27 February–2 March 1997. https://www.genome.gov/edkit/pdfs/1997a.pdf. Accessed December 9, 2017.

27. Wellcome Trust. Sharing data from large-scale biological research projects: report of Fort Lauderdale, FL, January 14–15, 2003 meeting. https://wellcome.ac.uk/sites/default/files/wtd003207_0.pdf. Accessed December 9, 2017.

28. Toronto International Data Release Workshop Authors. Prepublication data sharing [Opinion]. *Nature*. 2009;461(7261):168–170. doi: 10.1038/461168a.

29. National Institutes of Health. NIH genomic data sharing policy. https://osp.od.nih.gov/wp-content/uploads/NIH_GDS_Policy.pdf. Published August 27, 2014. Accessed December 9, 2017.

30. Bergen RP. Insurance coverage for clinical investigation. *JAMA*. 1967;201:305–306.

31. President's Commission for the Study of Ethical Problems in Medicine and Biomedical and Behavioral Research. *Report*. Washington, DC: US Government Printing Office; 1981. *Compensating for Research Injuries: The Ethical and Legal Implications of Programs to Redress Injured Subjects*. Vol 1. https://repository.library.georgetown.edu/handle/10822/559342. Accessed December 9, 2017.

32. Advisory Committee on Human Radiation Experiments. *The Human Radiation Experiments: Final Report of the President's Advisory Committee*. New York, NY: Oxford University Press; 1996.

33. National Bioethics Advisory Commission. *Report and Recommendations*. Bethesda, MD: National Bioethics Advisory Commission; 2001. *Ethical and Policy Issues in Research Involving Human Participants*. Vol 1. https://bioethicsarchive.georgetown.edu/nbac/human/overvol1.pdf. Accessed December 9, 2017.

34. Presidential Commission for the Study of Bioethical Issues. *Moral Science: Protecting Participants in Human Subjects Research*. Washington, DC: US Government Printing Office; 2010. https://bioethicsarchive.georgetown.edu/pcsbi/sites/default/files/Moral%20Science%20June%202012.pdf. Published December, 2011. Updated June, 2012. Accessed December 9, 2017.

35. Steinbrook R. Compensation for injured research subjects. *New England Journal of Medicine*. 2006;354(18):1871–1873.

36. Health Resources and Services Administration. National vaccine injury compensation program. http:/www.hrsa.gov/vaccine-compensation/index.html. Accessed December 9, 2017.

37. Remarks on accepting the report on the Advisory Committee on Human Radiation Experiments, October 3, 1995. In: *Public Papers of the Presidents: William*

J. Clinton, 1995, Book II, July 1 to December 31, 1995. Washington, DC: US Government Printing Office; 1995:1530–1532.

38. Hilts PJ. US to settle for $4.8 million in suits on radiation testing. *New York Times*. November 20, 1996. http://www.nytimes.com/1996/11/20/us/us-to-settle-for-4.8-million-in-suits-on-radiation-testing.html

39. C-SPAN. Human radiation experiments report of October 3, 1995. http://www.c-span.org/video/?67458-1/human-radiation-experiments-report. Accessed December 9, 2017.

40. Tavuchis N. *Mea Culpa: A Sociology of Apology and Reconciliation*. Palo Alto, CA: Stanford University Press; 1991.

41. Scher SJ, Darley JM. How effective are the things people say to apologize? Effects of the realization of the apology speech act. *Journal of Psycholinguistic Research*. 1997;26(1):127–140.

42. Remarks in apology to African-Americans on the Tuskegee Experiment, May 16, 1997. In: *Public Papers of the Presidents of the United States: William J. Clinton, January 1 to June 30, 1997*. Washington, DC: US Government Printing Office; 1997:607–609.

43. Centers for Disease Control and Prevention. The Tuskegee timeline. http://www.cdc.gov/tuskegee/timeline.htm. Accessed December 9, 2017.

44. Stein R. US apologizes for 1940s syphilis inoculation experiment in Guatemala. *Washington Post*. October 1, 2010. http://voices.washingtonpost.com/checkup/2010/10/us_apologizes_for_1940s_experi.html. Accessed December 9, 2017.

45. Reverby SM. "Normal exposure" and inoculation syphilis: a PHS "Tuskegee" doctor in Guatemala, 1946–1948. *Journal of Policy History*. 2011;23(1):6–28.

46. Presidential memorandum—review of human subjects protection [press release]. Washington, DC: The White House; November 24, 2010. https://www.whitehouse.gov/the-press-office/2010/11/24/presidential-memorandum-review-human-subjects-protection. Accessed December 9, 2017.

47. Presidential Commission for the Study of Bioethical Issues. *"Ethically Impossible": STD Research in Guatemala from 1946 to 1948*. Washington, DC: US Government Printing Office; 2011. https://bioethicsarchive.georgetown.edu/pcsbi/sites/default/files/Ethically%20Impossible%20(with%20linked%20historical%20documents)%202.7.13.pdf. Accessed December 9, 2017.

48. van Slyke CJ. New horizons in medical research. *Science*. 1946;104(2711):559–567.

49. Marston RQ. Medical science, the clinical trial, and society. *Hastings Center Report*. 1973;3(2):1–4.

50. Veatch RM. Human experimentation committees: professional or representative? *Hastings Center Report*. 1975;5(5):31–40.

51. Charo RA. Protecting us to death: women, pregnancy, and clinical research trials. *St. Louis Law Journal*. 1993;38(1):135–187.

52. NIH Revitalization Act of 1993, Pub L No. 103–143, 107 Stat 122.

53. US General Accounting Office. *Women's Health: FDA Needs to Ensure More Study of Gender in Prescription Drug Testing.* Washington, DC: US General Accounting Office; 1992. http://www.gao.gov/assets/220/216966.pdf. Accessed December 9, 2017.

54. Mastroianni AC, Faden R, Federman D, eds. *Women and Health Research: Ethical and Legal Issues of Including Women in Clinical Studies.* Vol 1. Washington, DC: National Academies Press; 1994.

55. Haas DM, Gallauresi B, Shields K, et al. Pharmacotherapy and pregnancy: highlights from the Third International Conference for Individualized Pharmacotherapy in Pregnancy. *Clinical Translational Science.* (2011)4(3):204–209.

56. National Institutes of Health. NIH policy and guidelines on the inclusion of children as participants in research involving human subjects. http://grants.nih.gov/grants/guide/notice-files/not98-024.html. Published March 6, 1998. Updated October 13, 2015. Accessed December 9, 2017.

57. National Institutes of Health. NIH policy and guidelines on the inclusion of women and minorities as subjects in clinical research—amended, October, 2001. https://grants.nih.gov/grants/funding/women_min/guidelines_amended_10_2001.htm. Accessed December 9, 2017.

58. Institute of Medicine. *Women's Health Research: Progress, Pitfalls and Promise.* Washington, DC: National Academies Press; 2010.

59. Meslin EM, Johnson S. National bioethics commissions and research ethics. In: Emanuel EJ, Grady C, Crouch RA, Lie RK, Miller FG, Wendler D, eds. *The Oxford Textbook of Clinical Research Ethics.* New York, NY: Oxford University Press; 2008:187–197.

60. Capron AM. The dog in the night-time: or, the curious relationship of the *Belmont Report* and the President's Commission. In: Childress JF, Meslin EM, Shapiro HT, eds. *Belmont Revisited: Ethical Principles for Research with Human Subjects.* Washington, DC: Georgetown University Press; 2005:29–40.

61. President's Commission for the Study of Ethical Problems in Medicine and Biomedical and Behavioral Research. *Protecting Human Subjects: The Adequacy and Uniformity of Federal Rules and their Implementation.* Washington, DC: US Government Printing Office; 1981. https://repository.library.georgetown.edu/handle/10822/559370. Accessed December 9, 2017.

62. President's Commission for the Study of Ethical Problems in Medicine and Biomedical and Behavioral Research. *Whistleblowing in Biomedical Research: Policies and Procedures for Responding to Reports of Misconduct.* Washington, DC: US Government Printing Office; 1981. https://repository.library.georgetown.edu/handle/10822/559380. Accessed December 9, 2017.

63. Faden RR, Mastroianni AC, Kahn JP. Beyond *Belmont:* trust, openness, and the work of the Advisory Committee on Human Radiation Experiments. In: Childress JF, Meslin EM, Shapiro HT, eds. *Belmont Revisited: Ethical Principles*

for Research with Human Subjects. Washington, DC: Georgetown University Press; 2005:41–54.

64. Childress JF, Meslin EM, Shapiro HT, eds. *Belmont Revisited: Ethical Principles for Research with Human Subjects.* Washington, DC: Georgetown University Press; 2005.

65. National Bioethics Advisory Commission. *Report and Recommendations.* Bethesda, MD: National Bioethics Advisory Commission; 1998. *Research Involving Persons with Mental Disorders That May Affect Their Decisionmaking Capacity.* Vol 1. https://bioethicsarchive.georgetown.edu/nbac/capacity/TOC. htm. Accessed December 9, 2017.

3 JUSTICE AND RESEARCH WITH THE VULNERABLE SICK

Baruch A. Brody
Neal W. Dickert

In recent years, the concept of justice in research has undergone an important shift. The older conceptualization, the protective conception, emphasized protection of vulnerable research subjects from being used in research without consent and from being exploited in risky research. The newer conceptualization, the balancing conception, more explicitly incorporates both access to potential benefits of research and population-based needs for research as additional demands of justice. Justice is now seen as demanding a balancing of access to research with protection from unconsented use and exploitation.

This chapter examines a number of examples of this reconceptualization in the context of research involving seriously ill patients for whom established therapies are unavailable or unsatisfactory. Many of these cases involve experimental therapies that are both promising and risky. The combination of need, therapeutic promise, consent-related challenges, and risk makes these patients both vulnerable to exploitation and in need of access to research. Each of these cases illustrates the importance and challenge of balancing justice-related demands, and each raises unique questions.

The first series of examples, involving research in acute, emergent illnesses, requires us to look at the impact of the balancing conception of justice on such fundamental commitments as that to informed consent. The second series of examples, involving research on new treatments for serious, but less-acute illnesses such as HIV and cancer, requires us to balance individuals' desire for access to emerging therapies and willingness to take risks with the social need for adequate evidence before drugs are approved for general use. The final example of Phase I oncology trials requires us to consider the implications of the balancing conception of justice on study design.

Research in Acute, Emergent Illnesses
Justice Over Time

The vulnerability of patients with acute, emergent conditions such as cardiac arrest, traumatic brain injury, stroke, and myocardial infarction is obvious. These conditions carry high risks of major impairment and death, and existing treatments for many of them remains suboptimal. These are also conditions in which carrying out an informed consent process is highly problematic or impossible. Patients are often unconscious or in distress, and surrogates are often unavailable within the timeframe during which trial enrollment must happen.

For years, no regulatory framework existed to allow such trials, with protective federal regulations only allowing research without prospective consent if risks to subjects were no more than minimal. Some studies did take place without prospective consent, often under a paradigm of "deferred consent" in which consent was sought after a patient regained capacity or a surrogate became available. However, in 1993, the US administrative office for research oversight officially determined deferred consent to be illegitimate and halted research in emergency settings unless prospective consent could be obtained or risks were minimal.[1] In 1996, US regulations were approved that allowed an exception from informed consent (EFIC) for research in emergency settings.[2] These regulations contain important provisions.[3] First, they require that prospective consent be impracticable (from patients or their surrogates) within the necessary therapeutic window of the intervention being studied. Second, the regulations require that the condition under study be life-threatening and that existing treatments are either unsatisfactory or unproven. Third, the study must offer subjects a potential for direct benefit, and the risks and benefits of the intervention under study must be "reasonable in relation to what is known about the medical condition of the potential class of subjects, the risks and benefits of standard therapy, if any, and what is known about the risks and benefits of the proposed intervention or activity" (21 CFR 50.24(a)(3)(iii)).[3] Finally, the regulations include requirements that investigators consult communities prior to study approval and publicly disclose the study's conduct and results.[4]

The EFIC regulations embrace the balancing concept of justice in important ways. Perhaps most importantly, they recognize the social need for research in emergency settings if treatments for acute conditions with high morbidity and mortality are to be improved. Also, the regulations explicitly require a potential for benefit and minimization of risk, though what constitutes reasonable risks or inadequacy of therapy can be a matter of interpretation and debate. Lastly, the requirement for community consultation represents a concrete attempt to understand public views of and concerns regarding the study prior to its implementation (see also Chapter 8). The Food and Drug Administration (FDA) does not specify which methods of consulting communities should be used, but it states that the process must provide an opportunity to discuss a proposed study with and solicit the opinions of the "community in which the study will take place and the community from which the study subjects will be drawn" (p. 25).[4] The results of community consultation must then be presented to an institutional review board (IRB) and considered in reviewing the protocol. This process is not intended to function as a consent replacement but rather to demonstrate respect for enrollees and communities and to make IRBs aware of potential concerns within the relevant communities. It may also serve important goals such as promoting trust in researchers and sharing responsibility for research conduct.[5-6] In these ways, the EFIC regulations concretely attempt to protect subjects and minimize exploitation while improving care for extremely vulnerable patients.

Although many investigators and IRBs must still become familiar with the EFIC regulations, there have been notable research successes since their passage. The Public Access Defibrillation Trial, for example, established the effectiveness of and resulted in the widespread availability of automated external defibrillators for cardiac arrest.[7-8] There have, however, been challenges and controversies that highlight the persistence and difficulty of justice-based issues associated with research in emergency settings.

In the early 2000s, Northfield Labs launched a multicenter Phase III trial of PolyHeme® (a polymerized hemoglobin blood substitute) in out-of-hospital victims of hemorrhagic shock, typically from traumatic injury. Because blood cannot be easily transported in ambulances, only intravenous fluid (which has no oxygen-carrying capacity) is generally given to these patients in the out-of-hospital setting. Patients in the trial were randomly assigned in the field to receive PolyHeme or normal saline. Upon hospital arrival, patients receiving PolyHeme continued to receive PolyHeme until they were successfully resuscitated, twelve hours had passed, or six units had been administered. Those assigned to saline received blood (standard therapy in hospitals).[9] While few disputed the importance of improving treatment for hemorrhagic shock in the field, the study unleashed significant controversy resulting in accusations from such prominent individuals as US Senator Charles Grassley (R-IA) that this study "makes the inhabitants of 32 communities in 18 states, and anyone living or traveling near these communities, potential 'guinea pigs' without their consent and, absent consent, without full awareness of the risks and benefits of the blood substitute."[10–11]

Much of the controversy centered on the in-hospital phase. Some ethicists argued that continued treatment with PolyHeme (under EFIC) after arrival in the hospital could not be justified because blood transfusion was neither unsatisfactory nor unproven.[12] Defenders countered that the known risks of transfusion rendered it unsatisfactory.[9,13] This debate is at the heart of concerns about protection in EFIC research; it illustrates the difficulty of defining what counts as a satisfactory treatment as well as what levels of risk are "reasonable" in the context of critical illness and no consent.[14]

Concerns were also expressed regarding the adequacy of community consultation and potential overrepresentation of minorities and economically disadvantaged individuals in the study. Particularly in light of reported low attendance and minimal minority representation in community consultation efforts at some sites, questions were raised about whether the interests and views of all community members were adequately represented.[15] In light of challenges in identifying and involving community members in these consultations, conceptual questions about the nature of community representation, and difficulty defining the relevant community, this study made clear the difficulty of carrying out the EFIC regulations.[14,16] These concerns had particular salience in the context of research that was being conducted in major urban centers. Questions were raised about whether this and other EFIC studies disproportionately enrolled poor and minority subjects; however, many conditions that are the subject of EFIC research, particularly traumatic injury, are particularly prevalent within these communities. What may appear to be disproportionate enrollment may actually reflect the distribution of the condition.[17–18]

Part of the PolyHeme legacy has been an increase in attention to and continued attempts to balance these justice-related concerns. The FDA solicited testimony from numerous stakeholders and experts and issued more guidance on community consultation in particular.[19] Investigators and IRBs continue to gain experience in evaluating EFIC proposals. And studies assessing the community consultation process as well as the views of enrolled subjects are helping to provide data to guide approaches to many concerns. However, important questions remain that call attention to fundamental tensions inherent in EFIC studies.

Looking Ahead

Perhaps the most obvious challenge for future research in emergency settings remains the community consultation requirement. In theory, community consultation holds promise in addressing justice issues. It offers an opportunity to learn about specific concerns potential research subjects have about a study, to take steps to address those concerns, to identify specific communities or patients who may want to be excluded, and to garner community-level support for a trial and thus share some responsibility for the trial's conduct. Community consultation is thus a potentially important way to advance protections and minimize exploitation. The PolyHeme controversy, however, reveals that operationalizing the requirement remains difficult.[14]

The challenge most directly connected to justice relates to the presence of dissenting views. Since passage of the EFIC regulations, many reports of community consultation results have been published. In these reports, "acceptance" of the proposed study and the EFIC mechanism have ranged from less than 50 percent to more than 90 percent.[20–23] The wording of questions and format of consultations both appear to affect measured acceptance,[21,24] but IRBs and investigators continue to struggle with what level of "acceptance" is enough. While cautions against treating community consultation as equivalent to a vote or "consent" are ubiquitous in federal guidance and the literature, the concept implies that there must be some level of objection within the community above which the balance is tipped and exception from "consent" becomes no longer justified.[4] This point has not been defined.

Real questions also exist regarding what constitutes adequate representation. Federal policy requires that community consultation involve both the geographic community where the study will be conducted and the community affected by the condition (individuals who have survived the condition, for example), but strategies vary for fulfilling this requirement. Some investigators conduct large surveys to represent a geographic area by quantitative means. Others conduct in-depth focus groups or meetings with key stakeholders including patients or civic leaders. These processes reflect very different goals and achieve different forms of "representation."

Defining acceptable risk in EFIC research also remains difficult. As illustrated by the PolyHeme controversy, divergent views exist regarding what constitutes "unsatisfactory" and "unproven" therapy, and it remains uncertain what benefits justify what risks in acute settings. These assessments are particularly critical regarding trials employing placebo designs or evaluating the removal of standard therapy.[4,14] For example, some scholars have raised concerns about the potential for cognitive harms associated with epinephrine use in cardiac arrest, an emergent condition for which consent to research partic-ipation is impracticable. There may become a need for a placebo-controlled trial of this cornerstone treatment in cardiac arrest to evaluate for the presence of harm.[25] What evidence needs to be present and what magni-tude of risk needs to be demonstrated before such a study is allowed is an area of uncertainty. Similarly, the range of acceptable use of placebo groups in EFIC research remains a challenge. As evidence mounts, placebo use begins to become more difficult to justify because of worries about depriving those assigned to the placebo group of potential benefits. These issues are challenging in any context, but the extent to which standards for uncer-tainty (equipoise) or risk/benefit balance are altered by absence of consent remains unclear.

A final important challenge is the category of patients who are conscious but for whom unavoidable barriers to consent are present. Paradigmatic conditions include stroke and myocardial infarction. In the case of stroke, patients are often impaired, and surrogates are typically asked for consent. While surrogates may be valuable in this setting, they are exposed to identical time constraints as patients, are likely under significant emotional stress, and are often unaware of research preferences of the patients for whom they are acting as surrogates.[26] In the case of myocardial infarction, patients are often in pain and distress but are capable of engaging in some conversation about potential enrollment. In both conditions, the EFIC mechanism is not typically used; however, complex decisions about enrollment must be made within minutes in situations characterized by mental and physical stress and signifi-cant risks associated with both action and inaction. In trials of treatments such as thrombolytic therapy (studied in myocardial infarction and stroke), for ex-ample, therapies may have significant risks and benefits, further complicating trial enrollment decisions.[27]

A small body of research suggests that research enrollment decisions in these acute contexts are largely uninformed, casting doubt on their legit-imacy and raising concerns about exploitation. Interestingly, there are also suggestions that patients want to be asked for permission and do not object to enrollment, though their understanding is often incomplete.[28-31] While EFIC enrollment may not be justified in many of these situations, consent processes may serve different functions than they do in other settings. That is, they may serve more to express respect and offer an opportunity to refuse than actually facilitate valid consent. The processes and forms, for example, that are required in standard contexts are thus probably not appropriate.[26,32] Unfortunately, there are no regulatory provisions that accommodate such situations.

There is an under-recognized continuum of potential involvement of acutely ill patients in research enrollment decisions. The current US regulations are binary; either a study is eligible for EFIC and additional protections are implemented, or it is not eligible for EFIC and consent is expected. Patients are not binary in this respect. Consistent with the balancing theory of justice that undergirds the EFIC regulations themselves, there is a need for a more subtle approach that carefully balances competing concerns in addition to ensuring rigorous scientific review.

Research with Patients with Poor Prognoses

Justice Over Time

There has been widespread recognition of the need to balance justice considerations in developing policy and practical approaches to development, testing, and approval of drugs, devices, and biologics.[27] Specifically, justice entails a requirement to balance protection of vulnerable potential subjects with the need to facilitate access to promising therapeutic agents for patients with poor prognoses and to protect the broader patient population against inefficacious and/or dangerous drugs. How these balances are struck has important implications regarding evidentiary requirements for safety and effectiveness, and consequently for study design. These issues have been central to difficult challenges regarding development of treatments for diseases such as HIV and cancer.

Since the policy reforms of the 1960s in response to the thalidomide tragedy, described in Chapter 6, new drugs are approved for use by national regulatory agencies only after their safety and efficacy have been demonstrated with scientific precision. Because the protective conception of justice was very influential, approval has historically been a rigorous and often lengthy process, even when new drugs are desperately needed. This emphasis on protection was challenged by AIDS activists in the 1980s who demanded quicker access to new drugs for what was then an essentially untreatable condition.[33-34] More recently, a 2010 New York Times article highlighted the case of two cousins with an aggressive melanoma (for which standard treatment is both toxic and minimally effective) who were randomly assigned to different arms of a Phase III trial of an investigational agent for which there were promising early-phase data.[35] The cousin assigned to conventional therapy died, and the case exposed deep tensions between the desire for rigorous randomized trials and the desire to optimally treat severely ill patients in contexts where standard treatment is known to be poor and patients are willing to forego the uncertainty of investigational agents for potential benefit that is otherwise unattainable.

The challenges are clear. Traditional randomized controlled trials (RCTs) can powerfully inform practice and policy by virtue of scientific strength and efficiency. Moreover, they avoid the kind of tragic outcomes seen in the 1990s with premature adoption of autologous bone marrow transplant for breast cancer. That therapy was adopted on a widespread basis based on early-phase evidence involving only surrogate markers (tumor shrinkage as opposed to survival) and led to numerous women receiving toxic treatment that was later shown to be nonbeneficial.[36] On the other hand, particularly in the face of promising early data and poor options, the merits of alternative research designs and the need to provide adequate care of current patients and potential subjects require serious consideration and balancing.

In recognition of these tensions, several programs have been adopted by the FDA. The Treatment Investigational New Drug (Treatment IND) program allows drugs to be used outside of clinical trials in treating immediately life-threatening (death is reasonably expected within months) or serious (not defined) illnesses provided that: "there is no comparable or satisfactory alternative drug or treatment available"; the drug is being investigated in controlled trials or all trials have been completed; and, the sponsor is actively pursuing marketing approval. Notably, FDA regulations are less restrictive regarding use in immediately life-threatening as opposed to serious conditions.[37-38]

The FDA has also enacted several specific mechanisms by which drug evaluation and approval can be expedited to facilitate general use, notably the Fast Track, Accelerated Approval, and Priority Review programs, along with the newly created Breakthrough Therapy designation.[38-39] These efforts are all designed to make the approval process faster and more efficient for drugs that show significant promise in treating "serious conditions," as defined by each program. Significantly, several of these processes accept surrogate endpoints (e.g., tumor shrinkage for cancer patients and improvements in CD4 counts for AIDS patients) that are thought to be predictive of clinical benefit as a basis for approval. It is often possible to collect data on surrogate endpoints much more quickly, and with fewer subjects, than to collect data on "hard" clinical endpoints such as survival or major morbidity, which may occur less frequently or take longer to occur. Importantly, because surrogate endpoints can be misleading, these programs contain requirements for sponsors to continue studies after approval to improve knowledge regarding safety and clinical efficacy.[40]

The spirit motivating these programs is well-illustrated in the following statement in the 1990 Final Report of the National Committee to Review

Current Procedures for Approval of New Drugs for Cancer and AIDS (the "Lasagna Report," so named for the committee's chair, Louis Lasagna):

> The committee recognizes that, by making new drugs available for marketing at this early stage, when there is substantial evidence but not yet definitive evidence of effectiveness, there is an attendant greater risk of serious adverse reactions that have not yet been discovered. Cancer and AIDS patients have made it clear to the committee, however, that in light of the seriousness of the diseases involved, they are willing to accept this greater risk. Earlier approval of new drugs will mean that the patient will bear greater responsibility, along with the physician, for understanding and accepting the risks involved (p. 3).[41]

The risks of early approval can be real. For example, antiarrhythmic drugs that were widely used to prevent ventricular arrhythmias after myocardial infarction were approved for use on the basis of their ability to suppress premature ventricular contractions (a surrogate endpoint for serious ventricular arrhythmias), but later were found in the Cardiac Arrhythmia Suppression Trial to actually increase mortality.[42] The notable shift represented in the expedited regulatory processes is the acceptance of some risk in exchange for improved access.

As in the case of research in the emergency setting, justice demands that no single value is treated as absolute, and that values be balanced. The accelerated regulatory approval processes are an attempt to do just that. After all, a policy that treated personal autonomy as an absolute value would abolish the need for official approval altogether, allowing official agencies at most to serve as information clearinghouses.[43-44] Alternatively, a policy designed to ensure protection alone would only allow approval of drugs with incontrovertible evidence of both efficacy and safety. Today, when there is promising evidence from trials, even from trials using surrogate endpoints, those who do not have other good treatments available are allowed take some chances with new treatments, provided adequate trial data continues to be collected to inform more complete assessments of clinical efficacy and safety. In this respect, these programs constitute an appropriate attempt to balance respecting personal autonomy and protecting patients in pursuit of justice in research.

Looking Ahead

The balancing act reflected in accelerated regulatory approval processes is far from complete and is not straightforward. Concerns have been raised regarding adequacy of postmarketing research for drugs approved on expedited tracks or based on surrogate endpoints. Some manufacturers, for example, have not adequately pursued postapproval studies necessary to justify regular approval after accelerated approval has been given.[45] Those failures can cause important harms and setbacks for patients, and some have argued that there is a need for greater enforcement of both conduct and rigor in the postapproval period.[46] Discussion is ongoing regarding what drugs should qualify for expedited tracks. What constitutes a "serious" condition is particularly ambiguous. Finally, it is important to ensure that clinicians understand the ways in which expedited approvals differ from conventional approvals. The evidence base for clinical safety and effectiveness may be weaker, and significant judgment may be needed regarding the proper clinical use of these agents.

Other relevant and important issues in the development and approval of new therapies for seriously ill patients include consideration of adaptive trial designs and efforts to harness the power of observational data. Adaptive designs, for example, are complex research designs that alter treatment assignment as a trial progresses and evidence builds. In this manner, they increase the chances of a participant being assigned to receive a beneficial therapy and may answer clinical questions more quickly with reduced exposure to inferior treatments. These designs may thus offer the potential for more refined balancing of justice considerations than traditional randomized controlled trials.[47] Similarly, further involvement of insurance companies and other payers in clinical trial design may help to ensure that trials meet endpoints that meaningfully inform coverage and resource allocation decisions. This was done, for example, in the case of lung-volume reduction surgery in severe emphysema through a linkage between the National Institutes of Health and the Center for Medicare and Medicaid Services.[48] All of these approaches involve attempts to balance competing considerations of justice.

Phase I Trials with Sick Patients

Justice Over Time

Phase I research is a particularly interesting and challenging stage of drug development and evaluation. The primary goal of a Phase I trial is to identify the maximum tolerated dose (MTD) of a new drug; it is not primarily designed to assess efficacy. Within oncology, the traditional approach is to administer the drug at a very low dose to an initial cohort of patients who have failed traditional therapy and then give increasing doses to later cohorts. Eventually, a dose is reached at which "dose-limiting toxicities" arise, and an MTD is determined. The MTD is then used in a subsequent Phase II preliminary efficacy trial. This is a primarily protective approach in that it emphasizes the safety of both Phase I and II cohorts by starting with low doses far below the predicted efficacious dose, thus minimizing exposure to potentially toxic doses.

Phase I trials for many conditions are conducted using participants who do not have the condition the drug is designed to treat because endpoints are pharmacokinetic and pharmacodynamics only (i.e., studying the interactions between the body and a drug). Phase I trials for cancer chemotherapeutic agents, however, are typically tested in patients who have failed other treatments. Because of these drugs' toxicity, it would be problematic to administer them to healthy subjects. This poses interesting justice-related challenges. Whereas healthy subjects have a vested interest in being exposed to minimally toxic agents, patients with refractory cancer have a strong (often primary) interest in receiving a dose most likely to be beneficial, even at the expense of greater risk of toxicity. A report from the M.D. Anderson Hospital of twenty-three published Phase I trials conducted in the period 1991–1993 found that in trials of drugs not previously tested in humans, a median of ten dose levels were required before the MTD was reached.[49] Moreover, the median resulting recommended dose was forty times the initial dose given, and almost one-third of patients in these trials received 70 percent less than the MTD. More recent reports have suggested closer to half of patients are receiving doses at or equivalent to the dose tested in Phase II studies, but it is clearly the case that subtherapeutic dosing is intrinsic to this design.[50] Estimates of therapeutic benefit in the context of traditional Phase I oncology trials have ranged widely, from 4–6 percent to almost 25 percent at six months of follow-up.[50–52] The variability may be largely attributable to whether surrogate measures such as "stability of disease" are characterized as true benefits when their clinical meaning or connection to the study drug is uncertain.[53] Regardless, most participants in traditional Phase I oncology trials do not derive clinical benefit from participation, many will receive subtherapeutic doses, and benefit may be more likely at the tail end of the trial (when the doses are higher) and will be affected by the choice of starting dose.

Those factors raise two connected ethical issues, both of which relate to the fact that the subjects are patients with life-threatening illnesses and few therapeutic options. The first has to do with informed consent. Are patient-subjects adequately informed about the realities (toxicities and likelihood of benefit) of these trials, particularly the potentially very different risk-benefit profiles at different stages of research? Second, is the standard Phase I design an appropriate balancing of the demands of protection and access?

At first glance, consent-related challenges in Phase I oncology research appear to be challenges of just that—consent—and not justice. However, because these challenges trace directly to these patients' illness and lack of treatment options, they contribute to concerns about exploitation and unjust distribution of risks. A growing body of evidence bolsters these concerns. One recent study of Phase I participants found that nearly 70 percent of subjects exhibited a therapeutic misconception, as measured by failure to recognize that research care is dictated by protocol and that the principal purpose of the study is to produce scientific information as opposed to clinical treatment.[54] That study, and others, also demonstrated significant mis-estimation of the likelihood of benefit (therapeutic mis-estimation) from Phase I participation, with 62 percent of patients estimating a greater than 70 percent chance of clinical benefit from participation, despite a historically low likelihood of benefit (less than 20 percent). And while more than a third of subjects expressed a desire to help others through participation, hope for benefit was the primary motivation in more than 90 percent of subjects. Interestingly, it has become increasingly recognized that some subjects' "mis-estimation" of potential benefits or misconceptions about purpose may instead reflect optimism or a "belief" that they will get better rather than an estimation of actual frequency of clinical improvement.[54–55] The extent to which such optimism or mis-estimation undermines consent—and the extent to which it is present in clinicians and researchers—is controversial, but there often appears to be a mismatch between study design and subjects' priorities.[56]

In contrast to EFIC studies, where regulations attempt to ensure a reasonable prospect of medical benefit for unconsenting subjects, Phase I research contains structural elements (dose-escalation) that minimize risk but also minimize the chance of benefit for early enrollees. There are multiple competing concerns that must be considered. Principally, participants' values and goals are highly relevant, and enrollment decisions may involve different goals.[56] For some, potential for benefit may be an overwhelming priority. For others, the presence of psychological benefit from "owning one's disease" or "doing something" in a way that coheres with the way they want to live their life may be particularly important. Still others may prioritize avoidance of toxicities that limit quality of life.[57]

The primary goal in minimizing exploitation is working to ensure that enrollment decisions are maximally consistent with patients' priorities. One important element of this approach must be a realistic and comprehensible presentation of research goals (including dose escalation), potential benefits, and risks. Clarifying the nature of the study design, and potentially the place of the patient in the dose-escalation plan, may help to make some of these issues clearer. Other strategies designed to help patients clarify (and communicate to physicians) their goals and values, to translate those values into participation decisions, and to ensure their awareness of palliative care options also play essential roles in minimizing exploitation and advancing justice. As described below, considerations of study design are also important.

In traditional Phase I dose-escalation designs, an acceptable risk-benefit ratio is sought primarily by protecting subjects from toxicities at the cost of lowering likelihood of receiving a therapeutic benefit. Several alternative approaches, however, have been advocated. One such method is the continual reassessment method (CRM).[58] Rather than starting with a minimally toxic dose, this method begins with the dosage anticipated to be recommended for study in the Phase II trial. Adjustments are made as toxicity data become available. This Bayesian approach (relying upon initial estimates of likely results) offers the hope of more responses, but at the price of more experienced toxicities. The resulting risk-benefit ratio, particularly at the beginning of the trial, may be more consistent with the goals of patients seeking enrollment in hope for direct benefit: access to potential benefit is emphasized more than protection from toxicities. Other proposed variations include allowing patients to choose among potential doses and employing more aggressive dose-escalation paradigms.[59] The largest review to date of alternative Phase I designs suggests that rates of benefit are relatively unchanged while rates of toxicities were higher in more aggressive dose-escalation paradigms.[50] However, Bayesian designs such as the CRM have not been specifically examined in this context and may offer more promise.

Looking Ahead

Vulnerable subjects should be protected from excessive toxicities. At the same time, they should have a better chance of access to dosages that are more likely to be effective. Society also has a need to complete Phase I trials as soon as possible so that trials of efficacy can begin. How to best balance these three goals in a proper trial design is unclear, although there are strong ethical reasons to advocate for and continue to explore less protective approaches for sick patients given what motivates most subjects to volunteer.

The traditional design of Phase I trials in oncology views dying patients as vulnerable and as requiring protection. This is reflected in the conservative choice of the initial dose and of the successive doses. Arguably, some dose-escalation designs may be too conservative, may not distribute potential for benefit or risk evenly across participants, and may not match expectations about the potential for direct benefit within Phase I studies. An ideal approach would optimally balance protection with assuring access to promising therapies, both for those in the Phase I trials and for those who will be enrolled in the succeeding Phase II and Phase III trials.

Conclusion

This chapter highlights some of the successes of the relatively recent reconceptualization of justice in research from a concept principally concerned with protection to one that balances multiple competing considerations. Justice must explicitly account for the value of protecting subjects, of respecting those subjects' goals, of promoting access to novel therapies in the context of severe illness, and of meeting the social need for research to advance care for the general population.

This conception of justice has led to better standards for research in emergency settings and consequently into improvements in clinical care for some severe, acute illnesses. It has led to valuable programs within the FDA to promote accelerated review and approval of therapies for serious but inadequately treated conditions. And it has driven a more subtle appreciation of the challenges of traditional Phase I oncology research, including a search for ethically optimized study designs. Major challenges in each of these areas remain, but this reconceptualization has represented a very important advance with tangible improvements.

Notes

1. Biros MH, Lewis RJ, Olson CM, Runge JW, Cummins RO, Fost N. Informed consent in emergency research: consensus statement from the Coalition Conference of Acute Resuscitation and Critical Care Researchers. *JAMA*. 1995;273(16):1283–1287.
2. Biros MH, Runge JW, Lewis RJ, Doherty C. Emergency medicine and the development of the Food and Drug Administration's final rule on informed consent and waiver of informed consent in emergency research circumstances. *Academic Emergency Medicine*. 1998;5(4):359–368.
3. US Food and Drug Administration. Protection of human subjects: exception from informed consent requirements for emergency research. 21 CFR §50.24(c). http://www.accessdata.fda.gov/scripts/cdrh/cfdocs/cfcfr/cfrsearch.cfm?fr=50.24. Accessed December 9, 2017.
4. US Food and Drug Administration. Guidance for institutional review boards, clinical investigators, and sponsors: exception from informed consent requirements for emergency research. http://www.fda.gov/downloads/RegulatoryInformation/Guidances/UCM249673.pdf. Published March 2011. Updated April 2013. Accessed December 9, 2017.

5. Dickert N, Sugarman J. Ethical goals of community consultation in research. *American Journal of Public Health.* 2005;95(7):1123–1127.

6. Richardson LD, Rhodes R, Ragin DF, Wilets I. The role of community consultation in the ethical conduct of research without consent. *American Journal of Bioethics.* 2006;6(3):33–35, discussion W46–W50.

7. Hallstrom AP, Ornato JP, Weisfeldt M, et al. Public-access defibrillation and survival after out-of-hospital cardiac arrest. *New England Journal of Medicine.* 2004;351(7):637–646.

8. Mosesso VN Jr, Brown LH, Greene HL, et al. Conducting research using the emergency exception from informed consent: the Public Access Defibrillation (PAD) Trial experience. *Resuscitation.* 2004;61(1):29–36.

9. Moore EE, Moore FA, Fabian TC, et al. Human polymerized hemoglobin for the treatment of hemorrhagic shock when blood is unavailable: the USA multicenter trial. *Journal of the American College of Surgeons.* 2009;208(1):1–13.

10. United States Senate Committee on Finance. Grassley: FDA needs to consider concerns of Human Research Protection Agency in blood substitute study [Newsroom]. March 13, 2006. http://www.finance.senate.gov/chairmans-news/grassley-fda-needs-to-consider-concerns-of-human-research-protection-agency-in-blood-substitute-study. Accessed December 9, 2017.

11. Grassley C. Americans should not be on a game show in emergency rooms and ambulances. *American Journal of Bioethics.* 2010;10(10):9–10.

12. Kipnis K, King NMP, Nelson RM. An open letter to institutional review boards considering Northfield Laboratories' PolyHeme® trial. *American Journal of Bioethics.* 2006;6(3):18–21.

13. Gould SA, Moore EE, Hoyt DB, et al. The life-sustaining capacity of human polymerized hemoglobin when red cells might be unavailable. *Journal of the American College of Surgeons.* 2002;195(4):445–452.

14. Dickert N, Sugarman J. Getting the ethics right regarding research in the emergency setting: lessons from the PolyHeme study. *Kennedy Institute of Ethics Journal.* 2007;17(2):153–169.

15. Holloway KFC. Accidental communities: race, emergency medicine, and the problem of PolyHeme®. *American Journal of Bioethics.* 2006;6(3):7–17.

16. Dickert NW, Sugarman J. Community consultation: not the problem—an important part of the solution. *American Journal of Bioethics.* 2006;6(3):26–28.

17. Sugarman J, Sitlani C, Andrusiek D, et al. Is the enrollment of racial and ethnic minorities in research in the emergency setting equitable? *Resuscitation.* 2009;80(6):644–649.

18. Clifton GL, Knudson P, McDonald M. Waiver of consent in studies of acute brain injury. *Journal of Neurotrauma.* 2002;19(10):1121–1126.

19. Biros MH. Struggling with the rule: the exception from informed consent in resuscitation research. *Academic Emergency Medicine.* 2007;14(4):344–345.

20. Biros MH, Sargent C, Miller K. Community attitudes towards emergency research and exception from informed consent. *Resuscitation.* 2009;80(12):1382–1387.

21. Dickert N, Mah VA, Biros MH, et al. Consulting communities when patients cannot consent: a multicenter study of community consultation for research in emergency settings. *Critical Care Medicine.* 2014;42(2):272–280.

22. Bulger EM, Schmidt TA, Cook AJ, et al. The random dialing survey as a tool for community consultation for research involving the emergency medicine exception from informed consent. *Annals of Emergency Medicine.* 2009;53(3):341–350.

23. Govindarajan P, Dickert NW, Meeker M, et al. Emergency research: using exception from informed consent, evaluation of community consultations. *Academic Emergency Medicine.* 2013;20(1):98–103.

24. Contant C, McCullough LB, Mangus L, Robertson C, Valadka A, Brody B. Community consultation in emergency research. *Critical Care Medicine.* 2006;34(8):2049–2052.

25. Hagihara A, Hasegawa M, Abe T, Nagata T, Wakata Y, Miyazaki S. Prehospital epinephrine use and survival among patients with out-of-hospital cardiac arrest. *JAMA.* 2012;307(11):1161–1168.

26. Dickert NW, Llanos A, Samady H. Re-visiting consent for clinical research on acute myocardial infarction and other emergent conditions. *Progress in Cardiovascular Diseases.* 2012;55(3):251–257.

27. Brody BA. *Ethical Issues in Drug Testing, Approval, and Pricing: The Clot-Dissolving Drugs.* New York, NY: Oxford University Press; 1995.

28. Gammelgaard A, Mortensen OS, Rossel PH; DANAMI-2 investigators. Patients' perceptions of informed consent in acute myocardial infarction research: a questionnaire-based survey of the consent process in the DANAMI-2 trial. *Heart.* 2004;90(10):1124–1128.

29. Gammelgaard A, Rossel P, Mortensen O; DANAMI-2 Investigators. Patients' perceptions of informed consent in acute myocardial infarction research: a Danish study. *Social Science & Medicine.* 2004;58(11):2313–2324.

30. Yuval R, Halon D, Merdler A, et al. Patient comprehension and reaction to participating in a double-blind randomized clinical trial (ISIS-4) in acute myocardial infarction. *Archives of Internal Medicine.* 2000;160(8):1142–1146.

31. Ågard A, Hermerén G, Herlitz J. Patients' experiences of intervention trials on the treatment of myocardial infarction: is it time to adjust the informed consent procedure to the patient's capacity? *Heart.* 2001;86(6):632–637.

32. Gammelgaard A. Informed consent in acute myocardial infarction research. *Journal of Medicine & Philosophy.* 2004;29(4):417–434.

33. Levine C. Has AIDS changed the ethics of human subjects research? *Journal of Law, Medicine & Health Care.* 1988;16(3–4):167–173.

34. Levine C, Dubler NN, Levine RJ. Building a new consensus: ethical principles and policies for clinical research on HIV/AIDS. *IRB: A Review of Human Subjects Research.* 1991;13(1–2):1–17.

35. Harmon A. New drugs stir debate on rules of clinical trials. *New York Times.* September 19, 2010;A1.

36. Mello MM, Brennan TA. The controversy over high-dose chemotherapy with autologous bone marrow transplant for breast cancer. *Health Affairs.* 2001;20(5):101–117.

37. US Food and Drug Administration. Drugs for human use: investigational new drug application (IND). 21 CFR §312.34-312.35 (2009). https://www.gpo.gov/fdsys/pkg/CFR-2009-title21-vol5/xml/CFR-2009-title21-vol5-part312-subpartB.xml. Accessed December 9, 2017.

38. US Food and Drug Administration. Treatment use of investigational drugs–information sheet. http://www.fda.gov/RegulatoryInformation/Guidances/ucm126495.htm. Updated January 19, 2016. Accessed December 9, 2017.

39. US Food and Drug Administration. Draft guidance for industry expedited programs for serious conditions–drugs and biologics; availability. *Federal Register.* 2013;78(123):38348–38349.

40. Fleming TR. Surrogate endpoints and FDA's accelerated approval process. *Health Affairs.* 2005;24(1):67–78.

41. President's Cancer Panel. *Final Report of the National Committee to Review Current Procedures for Approval of New Drugs for Cancer and AIDS.* Washington, DC: National Cancer Institute; 1990.

42. Temple R, Goldkind SF. The Food and Drug Administration and drug development: historic, scientific, and ethical considerations. In: Emanuel EJ, Grady C, Crouch RA, Lie RK, Miller FG, Wendler D, eds. *The Oxford Textbook of Clinical Research Ethics.* New York, NY: Oxford University Press; 2008:577–588.

43. Grabowski HG, Vernon JM. *The Regulation of Pharmaceuticals: Balancing the Benefits and Risks.* Washington, DC: American Enterprise Institute; 1983.

44. Green DG. Medicines in the marketplace: a study of safety regulation and price control in the supply of prescription medicines. *Institute of Economic Affairs Health Unit Papers.* 1987;(1).

45. Dhruva SS, Redberg RF. Accelerated approval and possible withdrawal of midodrine. *JAMA.* 2010;304(19):2172–2173.

46. Kramer DB, Kesselheim AS. User fees and beyond–the FDA Safety and Innovation Act of 2012. *New England Journal of Medicine.* 2012;367(14):1277–1279.

47. Truog RD. Randomized controlled trials: lessons from ECMO. *Clinical Research.* 1992;40(3):519–527.

48. Carino T, Sheingold S, Tunis S. Using clinical trials as a condition of coverage: lessons from the National Emphysema Treatment Trial. *Clinical Trials.* 2004;1(1):108–121.

49. Smith TL, Lee JJ, Kantarjian HM, Legha SS, Raber MN. Design and results of phase I cancer clinical trials: three-year experience at M.D. Anderson Cancer Center. *Journal of Clinical Oncology.* 1996;14(1):287–295.
50. Koyfman SA, Agrawal M, Garrett-Mayer E, et al. Risks and benefits associated with novel phase 1 oncology trial designs. *Cancer.* 2007;110(5):1115–1124.
51. Daugherty C, Ratain MJ, Grochowski E, et al. Perceptions of cancer patients and their physicians involved in phase I trials. *Journal of Clinical Oncology.* 1995;13(5):1062–1072.
52. Horstmann E, McCabe MS, Grochow L, et al. Risks and benefits of phase I oncology trials, 1991 through 2002. *New England Journal of Medicine.* 2005;352(9):895–904.
53. Miller FG, Joffe S. Benefit in phase 1 oncology trials: therapeutic misconception or reasonable treatment option? *Clinical Trials.* 2008;5(6):617–623.
54. Pentz RD, White M, Harvey RD, et al. Therapeutic misconception, misestimation, and optimism in participants enrolled in phase 1 trials. *Cancer.* 2012;118(18):4571–4578.
55. Weinfurt KP, Seils DM, Lin L, et al. Research participants' high expectations of benefit in early-phase oncology trials: are we asking the right question? *Journal of Clinical Oncology.* 2012;30(35):4396–4400.
56. Miller FG, Joffe S. Phase 1 oncology trials and informed consent. *Journal of Medical Ethics.* 2012;39(12):761–764.
57. Merritt M. Moral conflict in clinical trials. *Ethics.* 2005;115(2):306–330.
58. O'Quigley J, Pepe M, Fisher L. Continual reassessment method: a practical design for phase 1 clinical trials in cancer. *Biometrics.* 1990;46(1):33–48.
59. Daugherty CK, Ratain MJ, Minami H, et al. Study of cohort-specific consent and patient control in phase I cancer trials. *Journal of Clinical Oncology.* 1998;16(7):2305–2312.

4 JUSTICE AND RESEARCH IN POPULATIONS WITH COGNITIVE IMPAIRMENT

Scott Kim

Cognitive impairment is a general term that can include various neurodegenerative diseases (such as Alzheimer disease), acute confusional states (delirium), and impairments due to injury or stroke, among others. This chapter will examine issues arising from research involving persons with progressive loss of cognitive function, with Alzheimer disease (AD) as the main focus. AD is by far the most common cause of chronic and progressive loss of cognitive function. It is currently incurable, invariably leading to total disability and death. Nearly 14 percent of adults over the age of seventy suffer from some form of chronic and serious loss of cognitive function in the United States. Of these, 70 percent have AD.[1] Thus it is not surprising that there is an intense effort to find effective approaches to prevention and treatment for AD.

Dementia research requires participation of persons with significant cognitive impairment who may be unable to provide informed consent.[2,3] The loss of cognitive function not only leads to the loss of one's capacity to consent but also limits the ability to protect one's own welfare. As discussed in greater detail below, historically, persons with decisional impairment have been subject to some of the most notorious instances of unjust treatment of vulnerable persons in research. Indeed, concerns over violations of justice—through the exploitation of vulnerable, defenseless persons for the purported benefit of others—have been at the heart of ethical concern over the involvement of decisionally impaired persons in research.

Despite several decades of discussion, there is as yet no uniform policy regarding the involvement of decisionally impaired adults in clinical research in the United States.[4] While there are dedicated subparts to the federal regulations applicable to research with prisoners, pregnant women and fetuses, and children, there are not similar provisions for adults with decisional impairment. The regulations in principle do allow research involving decisionally incapable persons to proceed with third-party consent through a "legally authorized representative" (LAR) (§46.102(c)).[5] But the regulations defer to states and local jurisdictions for the definition of LAR, and the lack of uniformity results in potential uncertainty and confusion about who can serve as an LAR and the extent of the LAR's duties and responsibilities. In addition, although the regulations mention "mentally disabled persons" as a category for special attention in regard to subject recruitment (§46.111(a)(3))[5] and voluntariness of participation (§46.111(b)),[5] no specific guidance regarding these issues is provided to institutional review boards (IRBs).

This situation of uncertainty is not unique to the United States, however. In the United Kingdom, for example, different laws may apply depending on the location and type of research involving persons with dementia.[6] Given the absence of uniform and clear policy, AD research centers[7,8] and research ethics review boards[9,10] vary significantly in their practices.

The ethics of involving cognitively impaired persons will continue to be discussed as neuroscience research receives increasing public attention. For example, President Obama's April 2013 announcement of the BRAIN (Brain Research through Advancement in Neurotechnologies) Initiative[11] was followed by a charge to the Presidential Commission for the Study of Bioethical Issues to study both the ethics of conducting neuroscientific research and the ethical implications of neuroscience. Subsequent discussions of the Presidential Commission make clear that the ethics of research involving persons whose neurocognitive functions are impaired remain an issue of concern.[12]

Justice Over Time

A Brief Historical Review

Persons with decisional impairment have been particularly vulnerable to exploitation in research. Among the twenty-two notorious examples of unethical research studies documented by Henry Beecher in 1966,[13] nine studies involved at least some subjects who were decisionally vulnerable. These included "mental defectives," young children, confused patients, unconscious patients, and the "mentally retarded."[13] In most of these studies, the subjects were experimented upon merely because they were a convenient group who were available and could not resist, not because the experimenters were trying to develop treatments for conditions experienced by the subjects or people like them (see Chapter 9).

Over time, efforts to develop legal mechanisms to oversee the involvement of such persons in research have attempted to answer whether it is ever ethically acceptable to involve persons who may not be able to exercise their own decision-making powers in research. If it is ethically acceptable to involve such persons in research, then under what circumstances and with what restrictions would such involvement be ethically acceptable? A brief review of the attempts to answer these questions is important because over the years the context and nature of decisional vulnerability have changed significantly and, because of this, the nature of the justice concerns have also evolved.

Ethical concerns about involving decisionally impaired persons in research arose in a specific, historically conditioned context.[14] As discussed below, the topic has been addressed by at least three high-level commission reports in the United States over the years. Initially, the National Research Act[15] directed the National Commission for the Protection of Human Subjects of Biomedical and Behavioral Research to focus on the "institutionalized mentally infirm."[16] As the phrase indicates, this concern was complex, encompassing vulnerabilities created not only by conditions causing someone to be "mentally infirm" but also the impact of institutionalization.[16] Thus, although the National Commission did use the term "senile" twice in its report, its report targeted populations with a different vulnerability profile than those currently recruited for dementia research (see below). That is, its main focus was on those with mental illness and "mental retardation" who were institutionalized.[16]

The National Commission's report on those "institutionalized as mentally infirm" was not incorporated into federal research regulations as were the commission's other reports.[17] This occurred reportedly because of multiple factors, including controversies surrounding the singling out of psychiatric inpatients for regulation (further stigmatizing an already stigmatized group) as well as proposals that added multiple regulatory procedures (such as requiring consent auditors in even low-risk research) beyond those contained in the original recommendations of the commission.[17-19] The next national bioethics commission—the President's Commission for the Study of Ethical Problems in Medicine and Biomedical and Behavioral Research (1980–1983)— attempted to influence the Department of Health, Education, and Welfare (a predecessor agency to the Department of Health and Human Services, DHHS) to implement the National Commission's recommendations, but this effort failed.[18]

In the 1990s, another national debate took place, precipitated in large part by two events. First, in *T. D. v. New York Department of Mental Health*, a New York State agency's policy of allowing the participation of decisionally impaired subjects in research (by means of surrogate consent) for research was invalidated by the courts.[20] Second, a University of California, Los Angeles "wash out" study on schizophrenia[21] (where patient-subjects diagnosed with schizophrenia were required as part of research participation to stop taking their medications) was eventually found to have deficient informed consent practices. A 1998 National Bioethics Advisory Commission (NBAC) report[22] as well as state-level efforts of the late 1990s in New York and Maryland grew out of the discussion surrounding these events.[23,24] There have been two DHHS secretary's advisory groups since then who have addressed this issue[25,26] but neither have led to new federal regulations.

A comprehensive review of state laws in 2008 found continuing variability and lack of clear applicable laws in most jurisdictions.[4] In fact, there are only three states (California,[27] Virginia,[28] and New Jersey[29]) that have specifically addressed research involving decisionally impaired adults by making use of concepts in US federal regulations—that is, making clear how their local laws complement the federal regulations. In most other states, there are older laws about human experimentation or laws applying to health-care situations whose implications for the modern research context are not clear. Thus, for most jurisdictions in the United States, researchers and their institutions perform their own policy analyses in applying various laws that may or may not be relevant.[30] As noted by law professor Richard Bonnie in 1997, but still applicable today, " . . . the protection of cognitively impaired subjects depends too heavily on the diverse ethical sensitivities of individual investigators and on the ad hoc responses of particular IRBs" (p. 105).[18]

Current Context

Whereas the discussion over "mentally infirm" largely arose out of abuses of institutionalized persons lacking decisional capacity who were involved in research not relevant to their primary condition, the current context of research involving the decisionally impaired—especially for dementia research—is quite different. The justice concerns raised by the current context are therefore different as well.

First, there is now wide agreement that decisionally incapable persons should not be involved in research that can adequately be performed with capable subjects.[18,22,31] This widely shared view is perhaps the single most important principle in addressing the injustice of using weak and vulnerable individuals in research studies by those in positions of power over them. That is, it prohibits the most egregious types of injustice exemplified in past abuses so well documented by Beecher. This principle would still allow needed research involving the decisionally impaired to be carried out, as long as their involvement is justified by scientific necessity. For example, attempts to develop interventions to alter the course of AD or treat the symptoms of AD require persons who clearly meet the criteria for having AD. Since decisional impairment is an early feature of the disease, it is inevitable that such research cannot be scientifically valid without the involvement of some persons whose decisional abilities are impaired.

It is important to note, however, that the principle of excluding decisionally impaired subjects from research that can be performed with persons without such disability, while providing a much needed protection against unjust treatment of such subjects, raises a new and unanticipated justice issue. Such a principle would uniformly exclude persons with decisional impairment who have a serious medical condition (for example, cancer) from research that holds the prospect of direct benefit to them. Some might see this result as unjust; in the name of promoting justice, it could have the effect of excluding a disabled population from a potentially beneficial intervention.[32] Perhaps the principle of excluding decisionally impaired subjects from research that can be performed with persons without such impairment should be generally followed, but in unusual circumstances, when the potential for exploitation is outweighed by the potential for benefit, some exceptions could be made.

Second, the magnitude of the public health imperative is perhaps unprecedented, because the population of cognitively impaired elderly is rapidly expanding. Some estimate that AD will afflict 80.1 million people worldwide by 2040,[33] a staggering figure given that the illness invariably but slowly leads to total disability and death, causing not only immense suffering but also requiring tremendous public and private resources over protracted periods to care for those with the illness.[34] Given the relative lack of progress in developing effective treatments in combination with the devastating effects of the disease, even relatively invasive procedures with unpredictable risks have been approved and performed with AD subjects. Examples such as experimental studies with immune therapies and gene transfer neurosurgeries have resulted in serious harms arising from research procedures, such as permanent worsening of neurological status or even death.[35,36] Deep brain stimulation has also been investigated for the treatment of AD.[37]

Third, the decisionally incapacitated patient who is likely to be enrolled in clinical research today has a different vulnerability profile than those persons whose abuse originally began the public discussion of involving "mentally infirm" in clinical research. The specific context of AD clinical research generally involves outpatients living in the community (unless the intervention being tested is specifically aimed at those with more advanced diseases living in long-term care facilities). The population of concern in the 1970s—those mentally disabled institutionalized persons—were perhaps some of the most marginalized and neglected persons in our society. In contrast, today's participants of AD clinical research tend to be from sociodemographic backgrounds of relative privilege: There tends to be an overrepresentation of educated men from higher socioeconomic classes in AD clinical research.[38]

This is not to say that such persons are not vulnerable to unjust treatment. The point is that the vulnerability of the modern AD patient is one based more on *individual* vulnerability than on the vulnerabilities of a class of persons suffering societal inequities and neglect. More specifically, the vulnerability of the AD patient entering research today is one of whether he or she is being enrolled against his or her individual preferences or values. In contrast, the vulnerability of those who suffered research abuses documented by Beecher and others is one of those patients' incapacity being used as a convenient opportunity to benefit other groups in society.

Implications for Justice: Unresolved Issues

There is wide agreement that if we do not involve persons in research when they suffer from conditions that impair their decisional ability in research, then it will be difficult to develop the needed means to prevent, treat, or cure those very conditions that cause the incapacity. This would be a kind of injustice in itself, by abandoning entire classes of people on account of their "right to be protected." Yet, if enrolled in research, such persons remain vulnerable subjects due to their impairment. The kind of injustice that threatens the cognitively impaired research subject has shifted to one of individual vulnerability primarily based on the decisional impairment itself. Thus, the primary justice issue is the familiar one of how to balance the interests of the few research participants against the needs of society—but with the very important additional issue of achieving this balance when the research participants are too impaired to voluntarily give informed consent themselves. How can this balance be achieved? There are two main unresolved issues.

Who Should Be Allowed to Serve as the Decision-Maker for a Decisionally Incapable Potential Subject?

As noted before, although US federal regulations endorse the idea of informed consent by a LAR (§46.102(c), §46.116),[5] the regulations do not go much beyond this mere idea of third-party consent, and as described earlier, leave it to states and local jurisdictions to define who can serve as LAR. For most states where specific laws addressing surrogate consent for research do not exist, this may involve attempts to interpret statutes written for other purposes as applying to the research context. For example, for some types of "therapeutic" research, laws that permit *de facto* surrogates (i.e., not previously assigned as surrogates by the patient) to consent to *medical* (i.e., for the purposes of treatment, not research) procedures are sometimes put forward as permitting surrogate consent for research procedures. This seems to be within the bounds of interpretation allowed by the federal oversight office, the Office of Human Research Protections, in some instances[39,40] as well as by other sources,[22] although that does not guarantee that the individual states will interpret the laws the same way. The lack of consensus is reflected in practice. A 2002 survey of thirty AD Cooperative Study centers (which are funded by the National Institute on Aging) probably provides the best information available on the practices of AD researchers.[8] A majority (57 percent) of the centers reported using de facto family consent to enroll incapable subjects, 28 percent reported surrogate qualification that is more formal (such as power of attorney or guardianship), and 14 percent of sites reported that surrogate consent is not allowed. The clinical researchers' self-reports of their understanding of what is legally permitted in their jurisdictions, however, were often inaccurate (41 percent), perhaps reflecting the relatively uncertain state of policy in which institutions and researchers have developed their own local practices.

From a practical point of view, the central issue is whether and how to permit families and other intimates to serve as de facto surrogates or proxies (using the terms interchangeably for the purposes of this discussion). Advance directives (i.e., instructional directives) for research participation may be useful in certain contexts, but they are unlikely to be workable for many research studies, as discussed below. Also, while court-appointed guardians are often thought of as providing the highest level of legal protection for incapacitated persons, what is most legally protective does not necessarily translate into what is most ethical. For instance, unless the guardian is a known intimate of the subject, it is unlikely that he or she will have a reasonable basis to decide what the subject would have wanted. In research as in medical treatment settings, pragmatic and ethical considerations regarding surrogate consent lead to the following question: to what extent can a family member (as the most likely available and ethically defensible de facto surrogate) serve as a LAR for research purposes?

What Are Acceptable Levels of Risks and Potential Benefits?

The second major unresolved question for research based on surrogates' consent is *what are acceptable levels of risks and potential benefits?* Even if the designation of a LAR is clear, the issue of balancing the risks and burdens of research with the potential benefits (both to society and to the subject) remains. For instance, when the research has no prospect of potential direct medical benefit to the subjects, what is the highest level of risk and burden that should be allowed for such studies? In the pediatric setting, the line is drawn at "minor increase over minimal risk" with studies beyond that level of risk requiring a national level review (§46.406–407).[5] New Jersey and Virginia laws[28,29] on research with decisionally incapable adults use the same "minor increase over minimal" limit, whereas California law does not specify a level.[27] The most recent report on the topic, by the DHHS Secretary's Advisory Committee on Human Research Protections (2009), however, notes that "vitally important but ethically acceptable research would be prohibited by adopting 'minor increase over minimal risk' as upper limit of risk" and recommends a "soft cap" by using the term "moderate" level of risk as the limit (Rec. 5.h.2.b., n.11).[26]

The risk-benefit profile of a research protocol is important in another way. In general, the specific risk-benefit profile of a protocol should frame whether and how other related protections should be instituted. These may include, depending on the risk-benefit profile, addressing questions about how independent the capacity assessor should be from the research team, the level of rigor required in the assessment, the level of decisional abilities that ought to be present for the subject to be deemed capable, and whether other additional protections (e.g., consent monitors) should be instituted, among other issues.[30]

Public Perspectives: Family Surrogates and Acceptable Risks and Benefits

When the National Bioethics Advisory Commission published its 1998 report on the ethics of conducting research with decisionally impaired persons, there were few empirical studies to inform the commission's discussion.[22] Since then there has been a steadily increasing body of research that illuminates the two overarching unresolved issues regarding LARs and risk-benefit considerations.

Surveys of people at increased risk of AD,[41,42] elderly people in clinics and senior centers,[43] care providers of patients with dementia,[44] and the older general public[45] show that members in all these groups highly value AD research and many are willing to consider participation. Persons at increased risk for AD (due to age and family history) who volunteered for an AD prevention study, for example, were willing to be participants in AD research studies of varying risk-benefit profiles at rates comparable to or higher than their willingness to adopt a societal policy of allowing surrogate consent for such research studies.[42] In a nationally representative sample of US adults aged 51 years and older, 69 percent were willing to consider participation even in quite invasive experiments such as first-in-human neurosurgical gene transfer protocols for AD.[45]

Furthermore, people may be willing to give their future surrogates some or complete leeway regarding research participation decisions. The willingness to entrust wide decision-making authority to their future surrogates suggests that they value the role that their surrogates will play more than the specific preferences they currently hold.[41,43,45] Over one-quarter of the general population whose current wish is not to participate in future AD research also say that they would be willing to allow their future surrogates the leeway, if and when the time comes, to enroll them.[45] Among people who have first-degree relatives with AD, 80 percent state that their families could enroll them in potentially beneficial research even when their advance directive opposes enrollment in research.[41] This is not a paradox. People may be aware that their current preferences are speculative and thus value them less than their trust in the judgments of their loved ones who may have a more complete set of facts in the future.

The public's views on the ethics of dementia research have also been explored extensively using democratic deliberation (DD) methods that go beyond traditional surveys. As a method developed specifically for incorporating the public's considered views on complex policy issues, DD studies on research ethics issues provide an especially pertinent perspective on justice—that is, how the burdens and benefits of research should be balanced in our society. The practice of DD is built on normative theory that regards citizens' views as important and necessary resources for public policymaking. The goal is to obtain considered opinions of citizens that result from a fair, respectful, and transparent interchange of viewpoints based on thorough education and peer deliberation.[46,47] DD is increasingly recognized as useful for soliciting public opinion on controversial policies.[48–50]

In one study, members of the older general public participated in a daylong session of in-depth education and peer deliberation concerning the ethics of surrogate consent for dementia research.[51] There was broad initial support for a policy of surrogate consent for research—similar to findings from traditional surveys—that significantly increased further after deliberation.[52] A thorough qualitative analysis of the deliberations revealed an attitude of "cautious pragmatism" on the part of participants.[53] They demonstrated an awareness of both the pros and cons of policy options, while maintaining their focus on practical solutions. They were strongly attracted by the potential of advance directives but recognized their shortcomings and supported the need for surrogate consent for dementia research.[53]

The public's generally positive view of surrogate consent should not, however, be taken as unalloyed, idealistic trust in science. They recognize the potential pitfalls and their trust in the scientific enterprise and in surrogate decision-makers will likely fluctuate with how responsibly society manages the involvement of vulnerable, incapacitated subjects in research.[53]

Looking Ahead

We have thus far seen that the nature of justice concerns regarding persons with decisional impairment in research have changed over time. In the types of abuses documented by Beecher, we saw that persons with decisional impairment and incapacity were convenient groups for exploitation because they could not protect themselves. There is now widespread acceptance of the principle that, in general, decisionally impaired persons should only be enrolled in studies that concern those conditions that are causing their impairment. The cognitively impaired research subjects of today, when compared to those subjects who were exploited in institutional settings in the past, are vulnerable in a different way—mainly the vulnerability arising from the impairment itself rather than the setting. Thus, the core question of justice in research— how and to what extent should decisionally impaired persons be expected to bear research burdens and risks for the sake of the societal good of benefiting patients in the future—is mostly one of being sensitive to individual vulnerability rather than about protecting a class of persons. But as we have seen, providing clear policy on this topic has proved difficult, despite the widespread public support for family surrogate consent for AD research.

The remainder of this chapter will address two relatively neglected issues that may be helpful in future policy discussions: the limits of the distinction between capacity and incapacity, and concurrent proxy directives and preserved abilities. The focus of each examination is on ways to provide more evidence-based protections while decreasing the chances of unjustly excluding some persons from research participation and of erroneously including persons who should not be included.

Limits of the Distinction Between Capacity and Incapacity

Policy discussions usually do not take into account the reality that no clear-cut line exists between capacity and incapacity, at least when the decisional impairment is due to cognitive dysfunction (in contrast to, for example, incapacity due to delusions).[14] Thus, although some studies have found fairly good agreement among clinicians' judgments of patients' capacity,[2,54] others have found high rates of disagreement.[55-57] In one study, five experienced clinicians (from geriatric psychiatry, neurology and geriatric medicine) who evaluated the capacity of patients with mild AD achieved only 56 percent agreement.[56] In an experimental video survey that asked ninety-nine consulting psychiatrists to assess whether an AD subject portrayed on a video interview was capable of informed consent, 40 percent of respondents deemed the subject to be capable and the remainder deemed the subject to be incapable.[57] In another study, 555 capacity interviews of 188 patients with AD were evaluated by five experienced psychiatrists. For any given pair of psychiatrist judges, there was wide variation in judgments of capacity, and agreement ranged widely from slight to substantial.[58]

The early impact of AD on decisional capacity and the broad gray area between capacity and incapacity could have significant practical consequences. Suppose that for a neurosurgical gene transfer trial for AD it is decided that only patients who are competent to provide informed consent will be enrolled, owing to risk-benefit considerations. This is a theoretically reasonable approach but it relies on an assumption that it will be possible to enroll a sufficient number of patients with AD who are decisionally capable. For such a setting, the threshold for capacity would be set high[14,22] and, thus, only patients with an unequivocally high level of decision-making abilities would be deemed capable and thus eligible. But in a recent study of 188 patients with mild to moderate AD, less than 4 percent were judged to have the capacity to consent to a neurosurgical randomized controlled trial by all five clinicians who were shown the capacity interviews of the patients.[59] Furthermore, patients with such a high level of decision-making abilities may represent an atypical subgroup of those who have AD, raising issues concerning external validity. They would also have the most to lose from an adverse event, given their higher level of functioning. Finally, even though persons with AD could theoretically be deemed capable, their conditions still leave them vulnerable in other ways given their overall cognitive impairment. Thus, a normative position—developing practices based on the assumption of a bright line between capacity and incapacity—that is attractive in the abstract could be much less desirable when it is placed in context.

Concurrent Proxy Directives and Preserved Abilities

Since the idea of an advance directive is so attractive from a theoretical point of view (and is mentioned in most policy discussions), we need to address briefly why it is unlikely to be of practical value in this context. The rates of completion of research advance directives are likely to remain low.[41,60] Even among a highly motivated group of people—people already engaged in a clinical research study for first-degree relatives of patients with AD and most of whom expressed a willingness to complete advance directives—only 16 percent completed a research advance directive during the year following the survey.[41]

Even if advance directives are unlikely to be useful on a wide scale, however, it may be possible to develop a practice based on *concurrent* proxy directives that are completed *after* a person has already developed cognitive impairment but such impairment is mild enough to allow competent appointment of a proxy. A surrogate or proxy who is explicitly designated by the subject is ethically preferable to a *de facto* surrogate because such a designation expresses one of the most important values that the patient holds—who should represent his or her interests.[61] And, as we have seen above, the data on people's willingness to grant leeway to their future surrogates generally supports this view. A recent study found that over 90 percent of patients with AD in the early stages are capable of appointing a research proxy.[59] This suggests that for early-stage disease, a presumption of capacity to appoint a research proxy may be appropriate. Notably, 38 percent of those deemed incapable of consenting to a drug randomized controlled trial and 55 percent of those deemed incapable of consenting to a neurosurgical randomized controlled trial were still found to be capable of appointing a research proxy.[59] Thus, a substantial proportion of patients with AD who are incapable of research consent may be able to appoint a proxy in a concurrent rather than in an advance directive.[61]

Another ability that may be retained by a person with dementia is the ability to express preferences that are "reasonable"—for example, preferences that are consistent with the choices of people without impairments. Using hypothetical clinical vignettes for two major medical decisions (treatment decisions regarding a neoplasm and a cardiac condition), one study found that the treatment choices made by patients with AD did not differ from those made by healthy controls. Of course, the patients with AD performed significantly less well on measures of decision-making capacity but, notably, the content of their choice was not significantly different from that of the choices of the controls.[62] In another study using four research scenarios (drawing blood, a drug clinical trial, a drug challenge with PET scan, and a brain surgery study), patients with AD had similar participation preferences to controls for three (blood draw, PET study, and brain surgery) of the four research vignettes, with their willingness to participate declining as the risk increased.[63] The study also found that the more-impaired patients with AD are not more reckless than the less-impaired patients but, rather, are less willing to participate in research.[63] Another study has shown that patients with AD are able to discriminate between research scenarios with regard to whether they want proxy decision-making, and this desire varies according to the risk-benefit profile of the study; those who express reluctance to cede control furthermore cite desire for autonomy or study-specific features to explain their unwillingness, again indicating the presence of retained abilities.[64]

Thus, at least in the context of AD research, there is considerable evidence that focusing on the preserved abilities of potential research participants may provide creative avenues to addressing some difficult ethical issues. Among these, the possibility of developing a concurrent proxy directive holds great promise since such directives can be implemented at the time a proxy is needed. Further, evidence shows that even if people with dementia are not capable of independent informed consent, their preferences may still convey important information that can be used by their proxies, suggesting that a continued involvement of the impaired subject (as he or she is able) in decision-making should be the ideal. Given this evidence base, perhaps policies should reflect an approach that, while respecting the distinction between capacity and incapacity, provides a more reliable means of protection for these vulnerable persons, such as using concurrent proxy directives, being sensitive to subjects' remaining abilities, and providing guidance for their surrogates.[65]

Conclusion

Persons with cognitive dysfunction causing impaired decision-making abilities are highly vulnerable to unjust treatment because they are less able to make autonomous choices and to protect their own welfare. Historically, these vulnerabilities, in combination with social isolation and neglect of those with mental illness or "retardation", led to some of the most notorious cases of injustice in the history of human subject research. Those cases provided a key impetus to the development of the modern consensus: persons whose disorders impair their decisional abilities should in general only be involved in research that aims to address those disorders. This principle corrects the injustice of using groups of people as convenient research samples merely because they cannot protect themselves and not because it is scientifically necessary.

Despite this important progress there remains the question of how to justly balance the need to develop effective treatments for the public with the need to protect decisionally impaired adults in research when involving such persons is scientifically necessary. At least for dementia research, the context in which vulnerability due to decisional impairment must be addressed is now quite different from the original historical context. Indeed, the need for research, public support, and the widespread adoption of a human subject protection system have led to relatively stable, if not uniform, practices regarding how to conduct research with decisionally impaired subjects. However, the lack of clear policy regarding who can serve as a surrogate and how to incorporate risk-benefit analyses in such a policy continues to create an atmosphere of uncertainty for researchers and institutions, with the possibility that serious harms could still occur to research participants. Whether our society will be able to develop a set of uniform policies to remove such uncertainty and risk, without creating unwanted adverse consequences, remains a challenge. Given the increasing focus on brain research,[66] we may need more creative, context-based solutions to ensure that elderly, cognitively impaired persons are neither excluded from nor exploited in such research.

Notes

1. Plassman BL, Langa KM, Fisher GG, et al. Prevalence of dementia in the United States: the aging, demographics, and memory study. *Neuroepidemiology.* 2007;29(1–2):125–132.

2. Kim SYH, Caine ED, Currier GW, Leibovici A, Ryan JM. Assessing the competence of persons with Alzheimer's disease in providing informed consent for participation in research. *American Journal of Psychiatry.* 2001;158(5):712–717.

3. Okonkwo O, Griffith HR, Belue K, et al. Medical decision-making capacity in patients with mild cognitive impairment. *Neurology.* 2007;69(15):1528–1535.

4. Saks ER, Dunn LB, Wimer J, Gonzales M, Kim SYH. Proxy consent to research: the legal landscape. *Yale Journal of Health Law, Policy, and Ethics.* 2008;8(1):37–78.

5. US Department of Health and Human Services. Protection of human subjects. 45 CFR §46. http://www.hhs.gov/ohrp/regulations-and-policy/regulations/45-cfr-46/index.html. Revised January 15, 2009. Effective July 14, 2009. Accessed January 19, 2018.

6. Nuffield Council on Bioethics. *Dementia: Ethical Issues.* Cambridge, England: Cambridge Publishers; 2009.

7. Cahill M, Wichman A. Research involving persons with cognitive impairments: results of a survey of Alzheimer Disease research centers in the United States. *Alzheimer Disease & Associated Disorders.* 2000;14(1):20–27.

8. Karlawish JHT, Knopman D, Clark CM, et al. Informed consent for Alzheimer's Disease clinical trials: a survey of clinical investigators. *IRB: Ethics & Human Research*. 2002;24(5):1–5.

9. Gong MN, Winkel G, Rhodes R, Richardson LD, Silverstein JH. Surrogate consent for research involving adults with impaired decision making: survey of Institutional Review Board practices. *Critical Care Medicine*. 2010;38(11):2146–2154.

10. Bravo G, Dubois MF, Wildeman SM, et al. Research with decisionally incapacitated older adults: practices of Canadian research ethics boards. *IRB: Ethics & Human Research*. 2010;32(6):2–8.

11. Insel TR, Landis SC, Collins FS. The NIH BRAIN Initiative. *Science*. 2013;340(6133):687–688.

12. Presidential Commission for the Study of Bioethical Issues. *Gray Matters: Integrative Approaches for Neuroscience, Ethics, and Society*. Vol. 1. Washington, DC: US Government Printing Office; 2014. https://bioethicsarchive.georgetown.edu/pcsbi/node/3543.html. Accessed January 19, 2018.

13. Beecher HK. Ethics and clinical research. *New England Journal of Medicine*. 1966;274(24):1354–1360.

14. Kim SYH. *Evaluation of Capacity to Consent to Treatment and Research*. New York, NY: Oxford University Press; 2010.

15. National Research Act of 1974. Pub L No 93-348, 88 Stat 342.

16. National Commission for the Protection of Human Subjects of Biomedical and Behavioral Research. *Report and Recommendations*. Washington, DC: US Government Printing Office; 1978. *Research Involving Those Institutionalized as Mentally Infirm*, Vol. 1.

17. Levine RJ. *Ethics and Regulation of Clinical Research*. New Haven, CT: Yale University Press; 1986.

18. Bonnie R. Research with cognitively impaired subjects: unfinished business in the regulation of human research. *Archives of General Psychiatry*. 1997;54(2):105–111.

19. Berg JW. Legal and ethical complexities of consent with cognitively impaired research subjects: proposed guidelines. *Journal of Law, Medicine & Ethics*. 1996;24(1):18–35.

20. T.D. et al. v. New York State Office of Mental Health et al, 626 N.Y.S. 2d 1015 (N.Y. Sup. Ct. 1995).

21. Office for Protection from Research Risks. *Evaluation of Human Subject Protections in Schizophrenia Research Conducted by the University of California, Los Angeles*. Vol. 1. Washington, DC: US Department of Health and Human Services; 1994.

22. National Bioethics Advisory Commission. *Research Involving Persons with Mental Disorders That May Affect Their Decisionmaking Capacity*. Vol. 1. Bethesda, MD: National Bioethics Advisory Commission; 1998. https://bioethicsarchive.georgetown.edu/nbac/capacity/TOC.htm. Accessed January 19, 2018.

23. New York State Department of Health Advisory Work Group on Human Subject Research Involving Protected Classes. *Recommendations on the Oversight of Human Subject Research Involving the Protected Classes.* Albany, NY: State of New York Department of Health; 1998.

24. Workgroup on Research Involving Decisionally Incapacitated Subjects. *Final Report of the Attorney General's Research Working Group.* Annapolis, MD: Office of the Maryland Attorney General; 1998.

25. National Human Research Protections Advisory Committee. Report on informed consent and the decisionally impaired. http://wayback.archive-it.org/4657/20150930182942/http://www.hhs.gov/ohrp/archive/nhrpac/documents/nhrpac10.pdf. Accessed January 19, 2018.

26. Secretary's Advisory Committee on Human Research Protections. Recommendations Regarding Research Involving Individuals with Impaired Decision-making. http://www.hhs.gov/ohrp/sachrp-committee/recommendations/2009-july-15-letter-attachment/index.html. Accessed January 15, 2018.

27. California Health & Safety Code §24178 (amended 2002).

28. Human research, 32.1 VA Code §162.16-162.18 (2002).

29. Access to Medical Research Act, 26 NJ Code §14.1-14.5 (2008).

30. Kim SYH, Appelbaum PS, Jeste DV, Olin JT. Proxy and surrogate consent in geriatric neuropsychiatric research: update and recommendations. *American Journal of Psychiatry.* 2004;161(5):797–806.

31. Wendler D, Prasad K. Core safeguards for clinical research with adults who are unable to consent. *Annals of Internal Medicine.* 2001;135(7):514–523.

32. Shah SK, Persaud D, Wendler DS, et al. Research into a functional cure for HIV in neonates: the need for ethical foresight. *Lancet: Infectious Diseases.* 2014;14(9):893–898.

33. Ferri C, Prince M, Brayne C, et al. Global prevalence of dementia: a Delphi consensus study. *Lancet.* 2005;366(9503):2112–2117.

34. Hurd MD, Martorell P, Delavande A, Mullen KJ, Langa KM. Monetary costs of dementia in the United States. *New England Journal of Medicine.* 2013;368(14):1326–1334.

35. Orgogozo JM, Gilman S, Dartigues JF, et al. Subacute meningoencephalitis in a subset of patients with AD after Abeta42 immunization. *Neurology.* 2003;61(1):46–54.

36. Tuszynski MH, Thal L, Pay M, et al. A phase I clinical trial of nerve growth factor gene therapy for Alzheimer disease. *Nature Medicine.* 2005;11(5):551–555.

37. Smith GS, Laxton AW, Tang-Wai DF, et al. Increased cerebral metabolism after 1 year of deep brain stimulation in Alzheimer disease. *Archives of Neurology.* 2012;69(7):1141–1148.

38. Schneider LS, Olin JT, Lyness SA, Chui HC. Eligibility of Alzheimer's disease clinic patients for clinical trials. *Journal of the American Geriatrics Society.* 1997;45(8):923–928.

39. Office for Human Research Protections. Letter to Vanderbilt University/ Nashville Veterans Administration Medical Center re human research subject protections under Multiple Project Assurance (MPA) M-1363 dated February 4, 2002. http://archive.hhs.gov/ohrp/detrm_letrs/YR02/feb02h.pdf. Accessed October 28, 2016.

40. Office for Human Research Protections. Letter to Vanderbilt University/Nashville Veterans Administration Medical Center re human research subject protections under Multiple Project Assurance (MPA) M-1363 dated June 26, 2002. http://archive.hhs.gov/ohrp/detrm_letrs/YR02/jun02e.pdf. Accessed October 28, 2016.

41. Wendler D, Martinez RA, Fairclough D, Sunderland T, Emanuel E. Views of potential subjects toward proposed regulations for clinical research with adults unable to consent. *American Journal of Psychiatry*. 2002;159(4):585–591.

42. Kim SYH, Kim HM, McCallum C, Tariot PN. What do people at risk for Alzheimer's disease think about surrogate consent for research? *Neurology*. 2005;65(9):1395–1401.

43. Karlawish J, Rubright J, Casarett D, Cary M, Ten Have T, Sankar P. Older adults' attitudes toward enrollment of non-competent subjects participating in Alzheimer's research. *American Journal of Psychiatry*. 2009;166(2):131–134.

44. Kim SYH, Uhlmann RA, Appelbaum PS, et al. Deliberative assessment of surrogate consent in dementia research. *Alzheimer's and Dementia*. 2010;6(4):342–350.

45. Kim SY, Kim HM, Langa KM, Karlawish JH, Knopman DS, Appelbaum PS. Surrogate consent for dementia research: a national survey of older Americans. *Neurology*. 2009;72(2):149–155.

46. Fishkin JS. *The Voice of the People: Public Opinion and Democracy*. New Haven, CT: Yale University Press; 1997.

47. Freeman S. Deliberative democracy: a sympathetic comment. *Philosophy & Public Affairs*. 2000;29(4):371–419.

48. Mitton C, Smith N, Peacock S, Evoy B, Abelson J. Public participation in health care priority setting: a scoping review. *Health Policy*. 2009;91(3):219–228.

49. American Recovery and Reinvestment Act of 2009, Pub L No. 111-5, 123 Stat 115.

50. Presidential Commission for the Study of Bioethical Issues. *New Directions: The Ethics of Synthetic Biology and Emerging Technologies*. Washington, DC: US Government Printing Office; 2010. https://bioethicsarchive.georgetown.edu/pcsbi/synthetic-biology-report.html. Accessed Janauary 19, 2018.

51. Kim S, Wall I, Stanczyk A, De Vries R. Assessing the public's views in research ethics controversies: deliberative democracy and bioethics as natural allies. *Journal of Empirical Research on Human Research Ethics*. 2009;4(4):3–16.

52. Kim SYH, Kim HM, Knopman DS, De Vries R, Damschroder L, Appelbaum PS. Effect of public deliberation on attitudes toward surrogate consent for dementia research. *Neurology*. 2011;77(24):2097–2104.

53. DeVries RG, Ryan KA, Stanczyk A, et al. Public's approach to surrogate consent for dementia research: cautious pragmatism. *American Journal of Geriatric Psychiatry*. 2013;21(4):364–372.

54. Kim SYH, Appelbaum PS, Swan J, et al. Determining when impairment constitutes incapacity for informed consent in schizophrenia research. *British Journal of Psychiatry.* 2007;191(1):38–43.

55. Marson DC, Hawkins L, McInturff B, Harrell LE. Cognitive models that predict physician judgments of capacity to consent in mild Alzheimer's disease. *Journal of the American Geriatrics Society.* 1997;45(4):458–464.

56. Marson DC, McInturff B, Hawkins L, Bartolucci A, Harrell LE. Consistency of physician judgments of capacity to consent in mild Alzheimer's disease. *Journal of the American Geriatrics Society.* 1997;45(4):453–457.

57. Kim SYH, Caine ED, Swan JG, Appelbaum PS. Do clinicians follow a risk-sensitive model of capacity-determination? an experimental video survey. *Psychosomatics.* 2006;47(4):325–329.

58. Kim SYH, Appelbaum PS, Kim HM, et al. Variability of judgments of capacity: experience of capacity evaluators in a study of research consent capacity. *Psychosomatics.* 2011;52(4):346–353.

59. Kim SYH, Karlawish JH, Kim HM, Wall IF, Bozoki AC, Appelbaum PS. Preservation of the capacity to appoint a proxy decision maker: implications for dementia research. *Archives of General Psychiatry.* 2011;68(2):214–220.

60. Bravo G, Dubois M, Pâquet M. Advance directives for health care and research: prevalence and correlates. *Alzheimer Disease & Associated Disorders.* 2003;17(4):215–222.

61. Kim SYH, Appelbaum PS. The capacity to appoint a proxy and the possibility of concurrent proxy directives. *Behavioral Sciences & the Law.* 2006;24(4):469–478.

62. Marson DC, Ingram KK, Cody HA, Harrell LE. Assessing the competency of patients with Alzheimer's disease under different legal standards: a prototype instrument. *Archives of Neurology.* 1995;52(10):949–954.

63. Kim SYH, Cox C, Caine ED. Impaired decision-making ability in subjects with Alzheimer's disease and willingness to participate in research. *American Journal of Psychiatry.* 2002;159(5):797–802.

64. Stocking CB, Hougham GW, Danner DD, Patterson MB, Whitehouse PJ, Sachs GA. Speaking of research advance directives: planning for future research participation. *Neurology.* 2006;66(9):1361–1366.

65. Kim SYH. The ethics of informed consent in Alzheimer disease research. *Nature Reviews Neurology.* 2011;7(7):410–414.

66. Brain Research through Advancing Innovative Neurotechnologies (BRAIN) Working Group. *Brain 2025: A Scientific Vision.* Bethesda, MD: National Institutes of Health; 2014. https://www.braininitiative.nih.gov/pdf/BRAIN2025_508C.pdf. Accessed January 19, 2018.

5 JUSTICE AND PEDIATRIC RESEARCH

Lainie Friedman Ross
Robert M. Nelson

Striking the proper balance between excluding or including children in research is an ongoing challenge. Should policies and researchers exclude children from research participation so as to prevent potential harm to an individual child incapable of consent, or should they encourage participation and promote greater access to research so that an individual child may receive experimental therapy and/or advance the development of pediatric therapeutics? As we will show, in the latter half of the twentieth century, this balance swung from the exploitation of children to subsequent overprotection (or at least underinclusion). More recently, we have come to understand that children should be protected through, rather than from, research participation. This shift in the current balance of inclusion versus exclusion of children in research reveals changing conceptions of fairness and changing norms toward vulnerable populations.

Fairness in research can be evaluated by the distribution of benefits and burdens (e.g., risks) to children both as individual participants and as a class. An individual child may benefit from research participation in a variety of ways, including access to new experimental interventions, close monitoring, and/or evidence-based protocol-driven treatment. Children as a class benefit from prescribers knowing whether a drug is safe and effective for a specific pediatric indication. While an alternative to research participation may be to receive a currently available treatment that is marketed for adults, it may not be justified to assume that these off-label treatments are safer and/or more effective for children than an investigational intervention. Most drugs used to treat children have never been tested formally in children, making off-label use of medications the de facto standard of care in pediatrics in the United States and internationally.[1] In the 1990s, several studies found that approximately 75 percent of prescription medications listed in the *Physicians' Desk Reference* (PDR) lacked pediatric labeling.[2] An updated analysis of 2009 drug labeling found that the percentage of drugs with inadequate pediatric labeling had dropped to 54 percent.[3] The percentage of drugs that are used off-label, however, may vary when looking at the utilization of drugs in specific areas of pediatric practice. In a 2012 review, Kimland and Odlind found that the proportion of off-label drugs prescribed varied between 10 and 65 percent for pediatric and neonatal hospital inpatients, and between 11 and 31 percent for outpatients.[4] Thus, enrolling a child in a clinical trial may present a more favorable balance of risk and potential benefit than having the child treated by a clinician using a drug outside of its labeled indication or dosing instructions (i.e., off-label).

Inadequate prescribing information exposes children to unexpected adverse reactions or to suboptimal treatment.[5] Because children have not been sufficiently included in pharmaceutical research, adequate information may be lacking to guide the pediatric use of many commonly prescribed medications. As a result, any particular child is exposed to greater risk, and may be deprived of potential benefit, when compared to an adult given the same medication—an unfair difference based solely on age. This situation may be due to regulatory hurdles, economic disincentives, or reluctance to require pediatric studies unless the primary use of a drug will be in children.[6,7] The lack of an appropriate pediatric formulation of a drug may also deny a child access to an important therapeutic advance, or expose a child to a drug in one-off, poorly absorbed preparations. Also, the logistics of performing pediatric research may be more difficult given, for example, the lower incidence of a disease in children, the need for pediatric formulations, the need to stratify studies by age and/or weight to account for developmental differences, and the limited market for recapturing the costs of drug development.

In this chapter, we will review the historical role of children in research and examine the evolving policies regarding pharmaceutical testing that were often catalyzed by pediatric tragedy. We will also examine the evolving research regulations that govern the participation of children in biomedical and behavioral research based on the concepts of vulnerability, minimal risk, a minor increase over minimal risk, and prospect of direct benefit. After considering how the pendulum has swung from underprotection to overprotection (or at least restricted access), we evaluate whether the current balance in clinical research achieves an equitable distribution of benefits and burdens as required by justice as fairness.

Justice Over Time

A History of Exploitation

Prior to the twentieth century, children frequently were subjects in research because they were convenient: researchers would often experiment on their own children, servants, or slaves. Institutionalized children offered researchers a readily available pool of subjects whose environments could be tightly controlled. Children were also cheap and expendable, leading Lederer and Grodin to describe the history of children in medical research as largely one of child abuse.[8]

In 1966, Henry Beecher published his famous critique of failures in human subject protections in US research after World War II.[9] Of the twenty-two articles cited, four involved children, the most infamous of which was at the Willowbrook State School in New York City. It would be almost thirty years later before the US government publicly discussed human radiation experiments it conducted or funded during roughly that same period on the American population, including twenty-one experiments that specifically involved children.[10] One of the most egregious of these studies involved developmentally disabled youth who were institutionalized at the Walter E. Fernald State School outside Boston.

Willowbrook State School

A series of studies on infectious hepatitis were carried out at the Willowbrook State School from 1955 through the early 1970s. To understand the natural history and prevention of hepatitis, Saul Krugman and colleagues deliberately exposed a small group of newly admitted children to the endemic strain of hepatitis virus. This research design was justified, according to Krugman, given that (1) all the children would eventually contract hepatitis, (2) hepatitis was mild in this age group, (3) the deliberate infection might induce immunity to the endemic strain, (4) the children were isolated from other infections by being admitted to a special ward, and (5) only children whose parents consented were included.[11] In response to charges of exploiting cognitively disabled children, Krugman asserted that the fact that the children were cognitively disabled was relevant "only to the extent that society placed them in an institution where hepatitis was prevalent" (p. 160).[11] Further, Krugman maintained that neither he, his research staff, nor the staff of the institution were responsible for the "overcrowded, unhygienic conditions" at Willowbrook; rather, it was society that was responsible (p. 162).[11] Krugman also argued that "the overall risk for children in [the] special isolation unit was less than the risk for other children who were admitted to buildings in the institution where shigellosis and respiratory infections, as well as hepatitis, were endemic" (p. 161).[11] Thus, Krugman's main defense of the Willowbrook hepatitis experiments was that the risks of participation in research were no greater than, and arguably less than, the risks of everyday life for the children in this institutionalized population.

Theologian Paul Ramsey was one of the first to raise ethical concerns about the Willowbrook studies. Ramsey questioned the authority of any parent to enroll his or her child in a nontherapeutic study.[12] Even if such authority were granted, Ramsey felt that research should not be performed in "homes for the retarded because they are a captive population" (p. 41).[12] He detailed more specific criticisms as well. First, there was no attempt to enlist the adult staff in the research in spite of a similar risk of hepatitis. Second, there was no attempt to control the epidemic by "more ordinary, if more costly and less experimental, procedures" (p. 49).[12] The consequence is that "the special moral claims of children for care and protection are forgotten, and especially the claims of children who are most weak and vulnerable" (p. 51).[12] Finally, Ramsey criticized the letter that parents received offering possible admission into the hepatitis unit if they volunteer their child for the study as a clear example of coercion, arriving as it did days after a letter indicating the institution was full and their child was on a waiting list.[12] Suggesting that the children at Willowbrook were especially vulnerable to exploitation, Ramsey asked "whether the doctors would have accepted the hepatitis as a 'natural' occurrence and even as an opportunity for study" if Willowbrook "had been an orphanage for normal children or a floor of private patients, instead of a school for mentally defective children" (p. 49).[12]

David Rothman offered a similar critique: the fact that hepatitis was endemic to the institution neither justified the deliberate injection of infectious material nor qualified the study as a natural experiment.[13] He argued that "there is an essential difference between taking advantage of *social*, as opposed to biological, conditions" (p. 6);[13] "where the essential cause of a health problem is social deprivation, it is generally within the power of the research team to remedy the situation for their subjects" (p. 7).[13] Rothman concluded that the "Willowbrook experiment offer[s] both practical and principled support for maintaining as rigid a distinction between social deprivation and biological conditions as possible" (p. 6).[13]

Walter E. Fernald State School

In a report published in 1995, the US Advisory Committee on Human Radiation Experiments (ACHRE) examined twenty-one nontherapeutic studies using radioisotopes administered to children either conducted or funded by the federal government during the thirty years prior to 1974.[10] The only information available concerning parental authorization and subject selection for these studies is from a 1994 investigation by the Massachusetts Task Force on Human Subjects Research into research performed in 1946 and again between 1950 and

1953 at the Fernald State School. In a series of related experiments, one study exposed seventeen children to radioactive iron, while another exposed fifty-seven children to radioactive calcium. Letters to parents dated November 1949 and May 1953 failed to mention any risks associated with the research or the use of radioactive isotopes. Both letters implied that the research was intended for the child's benefit—an assertion that was false. The children who "voluntarily" enrolled into the studies were members of the school's so-called Science Club that provided special privileges in exchange for their participation. As with Willowbrook, the investigators at Fernald were not responsible for the living conditions and may have believed that the opportunity to participate in the research "brightened the lives of these children" (p. 346).[10] Nevertheless, "a particularly poignant dimension of the unfairness of using institutionalized children as subjects of research is that it permits investigators to secure cooperation by offering as special treats what other, noninstitutionalized children would find far less exceptional" (p. 345).[10] ACHRE concluded that, regardless of limited risk exposure, the children at Fernald were wronged by inadequate attention to parental permission and the lack of meaningful assent by the children—both made possible by their vulnerability and lack of social privilege.[10]

Observations

The studies at both the Willowbrook and Fernald schools involved children with developmental disabilities who were institutionalized. In both institutions, researchers unfairly took advantage of the social situations: overcrowding in Willowbrook made hepatitis endemic and social deprivation at Fernald made minor treats appear special. The fair selection of subjects is critical to avoid exploitation of a vulnerable group. While all children are vulnerable because they are dependent on others to consent or refuse to consent for their participation in research, developmentally disabled institutionalized children are more vulnerable because they belong to a group whose rights and interests have been socially disvalued.[14]

The abuses at Willowbrook and Fernald were not isolated events, as the reports by Beecher and the ACHRE document. We will discuss how public outcry in the early 1970s over research injustices spurred Congress to establish a national commission charged with developing regulations to protect human subjects in biomedical and behavioral research.

The History of Pharmaceutical Regulation

Today, pharmaceuticals must go through a rigorous approval process, with the requirement to demonstrate efficacy and safety before a drug can be licensed by the US Food and Drug Administration (FDA). This has not always been the case. The clamor for drug purity, safety, and efficacy only came about because of harms from unregulated medical products. Unfortunately, many of the events that stimulated legislation involved children as victims.

The history of drug safety and efficacy in the United States can be traced back to the 1848 Drug Importation Act which required US Customs Service inspection "to stop entry of tainted, low quality drugs from overseas" (p. 1).[15] More than fifty years would pass before Congress, in response to tragedy, would enact the Biologics Control Act of 1902 that was catalyzed by the deaths of thirteen children from tetanus-contaminated diphtheria antitoxin and nine children from contaminated smallpox vaccine. This act authorized issuance of regulations ensuring the safety, purity, and potency of vaccines, serums, toxins, antitoxins, and similar products.[16] In 1906, Congress passed the Food and Drugs Act that prohibited states from buying and selling food, drinks, and drugs that have been mislabeled and tainted.[15] However, the law was written narrowly and needed to be amended in 1912 to outlaw not just false and misleading statements about the ingredients or identity of a drug but also false medical claims.[15]

FDA recommended rewriting the 1906 Food and Drugs Act in 1933; however, it was only after the 1937 tragedy involving the antibiotic sulfanilamide (which was formulated in the poisonous liquid, diethylene glycol, and killed 107 persons, many of whom were children) that the 1938 federal Food, Drug, and Cosmetic Act (FDCA) was passed. It required "that new drugs show proof of safety."[15]

Voluntary reporting of drug reactions was started in 1952 after the FDA found that chloramphenicol, an antibiotic, caused nearly 180 cases of often deadly blood diseases such as aplastic anemia. Fetal malformations caused by the use of thalidomide in pregnant women led Congress to amend the FDCA in 1962 so that drugs not only had to be safe but also effective in the population for which they were marketed.[15,17] According to Chesney and Christensen, the unintended consequence of the 1962 amendment was to discourage "the evaluation of drugs in children because of perceived concerns over ethical issues, fears of 'harming' children and the perceived increased liability in 'testing' drugs in children" (p. 1129).[18] In effect, harms to children led to the societal benefit of established standards for demonstrating the safety and efficacy of drugs, yet the legislation had the unintended consequence of excluding children from reaping the benefits of those same standards—a clear violation of distributive justice.

Ironically, then, as FDA was taking on a greater role to ensure drug purity, safety, and efficacy, the pediatric community was expressing concern about the shift toward overprotection and thus exclusion from research. The term "therapeutic orphan" was coined by Harry Shirkey in 1968 to express the concern that children "have been denied the use of many new drugs" through the addition, since 1962, of a so-called orphaning clause that discouraged the pediatric use of new drugs (p. 119).[19] For example, many drug labels released since 1962 include phrases such as: "Not to be used in children" or "Not recommended for use in infants and young children since few studies have been conducted in this age group" or "Clinical studies have been insufficient to establish any recommendations for use in *infants* and *children*."[19] Thus, the lack of drug testing in children was leading to reduced access in the clinical setting to safe and effective medications.

US Research Regulations on Human Subject Protection

The National Research Act of 1974 was also passed, in part, in response to tragedy: the public awareness of the United States Public Health Service's research at Tuskegee, Alabama, which was an observational study of the natural progression of untreated syphilis in rural African American men who were deceived into participating and then had effective treatment (penicillin) withheld for decades. The 1974 act created the National Commission for the Protection of Human Subjects of Biomedical and Behavioral Research (hereinafter, the National Commission) that was authorized to identify the underlying basic ethical principles and develop guidelines for human subjects research, including research involving children.[20]

The National Commission published its landmark work on the basic ethical principles, the *Belmont Report*, in 1979. The *Belmont Report* interprets the principle of justice to require "fair procedures . . . [for] the selection of research subjects" so that persons are not included "simply because of their easy availability, their compromised position, or their manipulability" (pp. 23194, 23196).[21] Persons who are "vulnerable" to such exploitation are defined either as someone who is incapable of giving informed consent (e.g., children or the mentally infirm) or, if capable, who may not be positioned to give that consent voluntarily (e.g., prisoners). The capacity to give voluntary informed consent thus becomes part of the procedure by which justice is addressed—"it [is] a matter of social justice that there is an order of preference in the selection of classes of subjects (e.g., adults before children) and that some classes of potential subjects (e.g., the institutionalized mentally infirm or prisoners) may be involved as research subjects, if at all, only on certain conditions" (p. 23196).[21] These conditions require that the subject may personally benefit from the research or "the research is directly related to the specific conditions of the class involved" (p. 23197).[21] Thus, social justice requires a careful balancing between protecting children from unnecessary exposure to research risks (i.e., preferring adults) and providing access to investigational products so that the benefits (i.e., safety and efficacy) of these products *for children* can be established.

The National Commission proposed an equitable balance between participation and protection of children in research in a report entitled *Research Involving Children*[22] that proposed additional safeguards for children in research. This report served as the basis for the pediatric federal regulations, often referred to as Subpart D*[23,24]. Subpart D defines the limits of permissible pediatric research based on an assessment of risk and potential benefit. It also clarifies whose permission is needed for the child to participate in research, and the role for the child's assent.

Under subpart D, healthy children can participate in research provided that it exposes them to no more than minimal risk. In contrast, children with a disorder or condition can be exposed to a minor increase over minimal risk. If the research offers the prospect of direct benefit, then greater risk is tolerated, but the risks must be justified by the anticipated benefit, and the "relation of the anticipated benefit to the risk must be at least as favorable to the subjects as that presented by available alternative approaches."[23,24] Other research may be permissible, but it must be approved by a national review committee.[23,24]

Subpart D Research Categories

The National Commission introduced the concept of "minimal risk" to limit parental discretion regarding a child's research participation absent the potential for direct benefit to the child. Before allowing a parent to permit a child's participation, an institutional review board (IRB) must determine the extent to which the research presents risks commensurate with that child's situation. The federal regulations define "minimal risk" as "the probability and magnitude of harm or discomfort anticipated in the research are not greater in and of themselves than those ordinarily encountered in daily life or during the performance of routine physical or psychological examinations or tests."[23,24] This definition contrasts with the definition of minimal risk offered by the National Commission in that the phrase "of healthy children" is missing.[22] This creates an ambiguity in that the risks of research may be indexed to the "ordinary" experience of sick children rather than healthy children. Since sick children may be exposed to invasive medical interventions (e.g., lumbar

---

* The pediatric federal regulations were promulgated by: (1) the Department of Health and Human Services and codified at Title 45, part 46, Subpart D of the Code of Federal Regulations; and (2) the Food and Drug Administration and codified at Title 21, part 50, subpart D of the Code of Federal Regulations.

puncture), these procedures may be considered within their "ordinary experience" and thus minimal risk. This ambiguity also leaves open the possibility that children who live in crime-ridden areas could be exposed to greater risk in research because they are exposed to greater risk in their ordinary lives. Following the National Commission, three US–based advisory panels, the Institute of Medicine (IOM, now the National Academy of Medicine), the Secretary's Advisory Committee on Human Research Protections (SACHRP), and the National Human Research Protections Advisory Committee, have all recommended the use of a uniform standard for minimal risk indexed to normal healthy children.[25,26,27] And yet, data show that IRBs demonstrate wide variability in whether a given procedure or intervention meets the minimal risk threshold.[28] Whether this variability is a result of this ambiguity is not known.

Most ethicists also disagree with the nonuniform interpretation of minimal risk. Terrence Ackerman, for example, interprets activities that are "normally encountered by a child" not to mean any activity that a child may have previously experienced, but rather an activity with which the child is familiar and with which he is able to cope well: "The fact that a sick child has undergone a particular procedure, such as a lumbar puncture, during treatment does not guarantee that he or she will not be subjected to considerable stress or anxiety"(p. 4).[29] He has offered the following definition of minimal risk as an alternative:

A research procedure involving minimal risk is one in which the probability of physical and psychological harm is no more than that to which it is appropriate to intentionally expose a child for educational purposes in family life situations. (p. 106)[30]

This definition would be appropriate for healthy children, children with a disorder, and those at risk (i.e., with a condition) because, as Ross explains, "it allows parents to balance the responsibility of protecting their child from harm and promoting their child's moral development" (p. 85).[31] The argument that parents can morally permit their child to participate in research in order to promote the child's moral development was a concept originally proposed by William Bartholome.[32]

The National Commission also supported research interventions and/or procedures that present greater than minimal risk but where the risk is justified by the anticipated direct benefit to the enrolled children, and where the relation of the anticipated benefit to such risk is at least as favorable as that presented by available alternative approaches. The ethical justification of these two types of research was "straightforward" as an application of the ethical principle of beneficence (and the corollary to minimize harm), along with the view that exposure to minimal risk activities falls within the appropriate scope of parental responsibility. However, the National Commission was concerned that limiting research to these two categories would exclude important research. They developed an "escape hatch" that became the process of public review by a national advisory panel (p. 167).[33] The National Commission also proposed a fourth category of research to limit referrals to a national advisory panel: nonbeneficial research involving a minor increase over minimal risk if the research investigated a child's "disorder or condition."[22] This category presented the most controversy. The majority argument in favor of allowing children to participate in such research was largely pragmatic, based on "examples of diagnostic, therapeutic and preventive measures that might well have been derived from research involving risk that, while minor, would be considered more than minimal" (pp. 126–127).[22] (The National Commission also noted that "parental authority routinely covers a child's participation in many activities [such as skiing and contact sports] in which risk is more than minimal, and yet benefit is questionable" (p. 152)).[22] One dissenting commissioner, Robert Turtle, reflecting the ambiguity of indexing risk, characterized the majority argument as follows: first, sick children are subject to unique risks and experiences; second, added research "risks [should be] similar to the risks and experiences familiar to [sick] children" (p. 148);[22] finally, added research risks are normal for these children and thus should be permitted. The child's illness does not warrant additional protections, but rather is felt to be an appropriate difference on which to base exposure to greater than minimal risk. Against this majority view, Turtle argued that children who are exposed to greater risks due to their condition or treatment "cannot ethically be assumed to qualify for additional risk." In his estimate, such an argument perverts the anchoring of "minimal risk" to the "ordinary everyday risks of childhood."[22] The result will be to direct "researchers to involve more sick children as research subjects" in greater than minimal risk research, thus ignoring aggregate risks and placing the burden of research on the sick child "in clear violation of [the] principle of justice" (pp. 147–148).[22] Elsewhere we have proposed that all nonbeneficial research on children should be held to one level of risk on the grounds that when the research offers no prospect of direct benefit, justice requires that the risks are fairly and widely distributed.[34]

Vulnerability

The National Commission was particularly aware that some populations are more vulnerable than others, and sought to minimize the risks to which these groups were exposed. First, it proposed that research be done, when possible, first on animals, then adults followed by older children. Second, children who are wards of the state could only participate in research that was either related to their status as wards or conducted in settings such as schools, camps, hospitals, or institutions where the majority of enrolled children are not wards. Third, the National Commission addressed two additional vulnerable pediatric subpopulations: institutionalized children and children confined to correctional institutions. The National Commission argued that they should participate in research "only if the conditions regarding research on the institutionalized mentally infirm or on prisoners (as applicable) are fulfilled in addition to the criterion set forth herein" (pp. 19–20).[22]

The Willowbrook and Fernald studies were examples of the type of research that the current federal regulations governing research were designed to prevent. Appealing to the formal principle of justice (i.e., treating like cases alike), the condition of these children as both intellectually disabled and institutionalized should not count as a relevant difference in allowing them to be treated unequally. The condition of these children made them vulnerable to exploitation as research subjects and thereby exposure to an unfair share of research risk. The physicians involved claimed that participating in the research was to the advantage of the children being studied, an argument that appears compatible with the notion of justice as fairness. According to this understanding of justice, differences in treatment may be justified as long as the difference results in an overall advantage or benefit to the individual being studied.[35] However, exposing an "at-risk" child to increased risk or inducing a "deprived" child to participate through an otherwise meager benefit hardly seems fair, especially if the child's situation could have been improved through nonresearch interventions. Any justification of increased research risk exposure based on a child's "social" condition must be viewed critically through the lens of justice. On such a view, the institutional conditions that placed these children "at risk" should have been the target of corrective actions, rather than the background conditions that justified the unequal treatment.

The Shift to Access

Despite the passage of federal regulations in 1983 to guide researchers and those who provide research oversight (institutional review boards) regarding the participation of children in biomedical and behavioral research,[36] the underinclusion of children in some research, particularly drug research, led to a report by the American Academy of Pediatrics (AAP) Committee on Drugs in 1994 entitled "Guidelines for the Ethical Conduct of Studies to Evaluate

Drugs in Pediatric Populations"[37] The AAP policy statement cited the data that over 75 percent of medications listed in the *Physicians' Desk Reference* included a "disclaimer or lack of dose information for use by children" (p. 286).[37] Like Shirkey, the AAP Committee on Drugs objected to what they perceived as over-protection: "since implementation of the 1962 Kefauver-Harris amendments of the federal Food, Drug and Cosmetic Act, children have not shared in ther-apeutic advances to the same extent as adults" (p. 286).[37]

Beginning in the mid-1990s, there were numerous changes in legislation and policies to improve pediatric drug information. In 1994, FDA published specific requirements on the content and format of pediatric labeling for human prescription drugs.[38] FDA required drug manufacturers to survey ex-isting data and determine whether those data were sufficient to support addi-tional pediatric use information in drug labeling. Disappointingly, more than half of the manufacturers simply requested that the drug label include the phrase "Safety and effectiveness in pediatric patients have not been estab-lished" (p. 66632).[39]

In 1997, the FDA Modernization Act (FDAMA) was passed, encouraging pharmaceutical companies to perform pediatric studies for "on-patent" drugs to gain an extra six months of marketing exclusivity that can be worth millions and perhaps hundreds of millions of dollars.[40] This voluntary incentive was modified and re-enacted in 2002, 2007, and made permanent in 2012 as the Best Pharmaceuticals for Children Act (BPCA). BPCA also established a pro-cess at NIH for prioritizing and studying off-patent medicines, which was reauthorized in 2007, 2012, and again in 2017.[41,42,43] This off-patent process is an important addition because there is a predominance of off-patent drug use in the pediatric setting (with suggestions that it may account for as much as 70 percent of drugs used).[44]

In 1998, the FDA published the Pediatric Rule that required manufacturers of certain new drugs and biological products to conduct studies to provide ad-equate pediatric labeling based on the adult indication.[39] Enjoined in 2002 following a legal challenge that FDA had exceeded its statutory authority, the Rule was replaced by legislation entitled the Pediatric Research Equity Act (PREA) in November 2003.[45] PREA was renewed in 2007. The FDA Safety and Innovation Act of 2012 re-authorized PREA and BPCA, making permanent the requirement to conduct pediatric studies for certain new drugs and bio-logical products (PREA) and the voluntary marketing incentive for on-patent drugs (BPCA). It also renewed the NIH off-patent program for another five years, which was extended by the FDA Reauthorization Act of 2017 for another five years.[42,43] NIH also issued new policy guidelines in 1998 to increase the enrollment of children in research studies.[46] Analogous to the NIH policy in

1994 that required NIH–funded research to include women and minorities, the 1998 guidelines require the inclusion of children, unless there is good justification to exclude them.

The vulnerability of children based on their inability to consent for themselves serves as an appropriate justification for establishing additional protections when they are enrolled in research. However, protection must be balanced by access so that children do not fail to benefit from therapeutic advances. Many of the policies that promote access have been designed to maximize benefits to children as a class (i.e., ensuring the availability of treatment proven safe and effective for different age groups) while minimizing harm to individual children (i.e., by obviating the need for off-label usage).

What Have the New Legislation and Policies Achieved?

By 2017, BPCA and PREA have increased the participation of children in pharmaceutical research, resulting in 642 pediatric labeling changes as a result of new pediatric studies,[47] and pediatric exclusivity for 214 products.[48] Although the percentage of drugs with some pediatric labeling has increased from 22 percent in 1975 to 46 percent in 2009,[3] the impact of these legislative incentives on pediatric labeling for products used in clinical practice is mixed. For example, data from a pediatric intensive care unit in 2008 found that "67% of medications prescribed and administered in the pediatric intensive care unit did not have Food and Drug Administration approval or had only limited approval" (p. e195).[49] In 2012, Laughon and colleagues reported that "nine out of the ten most commonly used therapeutics in the neonatal intensive care units are not labeled for use in premature infants" (p. 644).[50] With respect to the studies encouraged under pediatric exclusivity, they note that "few have included infant-specific labeling. Infants (<1 year of age) and premature infants represent only 0.2 and 0.01%, respectively, of all children studies in trials submitted to the FDA through the pediatric exclusivity program in 1998–2005" (p. 644).[50] That is, while gaps exist for children of all ages, off-label usage of pharmaceuticals remains most severe in neonates.[51] Justice requires that we do not exclude one group (e.g., neonates), particularly if the treatment is necessary in infancy.

The development of appropriate pediatric formulations, especially for the use of off-patent drugs in infants and young children, remains a challenge. Milne found that of the more than 130 products studied to provide new pediatric labeling under BPCA, "as of mid-2007, only 8% had new pediatric formulations, while another 8% provided information on preparation of suspension or recipes for extemporaneous compounding" (p. 2135).[44] When BPCA was renewed in 2007, specific language was added encouraging the development and use of age-appropriate formulations. Another concern was that BPCA would only stimulate pediatric studies of blockbuster patent drugs, because the greater the financial gains for a particular drug, the more valuable an additional six months of exclusivity would be. However studies to date show this fear to be unfounded as the trials reflect pediatric disease burden.[52,53]

Has the NIH policy to increase the enrollment of children in adult studies achieved its goals? Permitting children to enroll in adult trials is not enough; rather, to justify the enrollment of children, the study design must include plans to analyze the data obtained from children and adults separately. Otherwise, the enrollment of children only helps to achieve overall accrual goals, and may not provide information that advances pediatric medicine. Failing to obtain useful pediatric data from the enrollment of children in research is contrary to the principle of justice that preferentially enrolls adults in research who can consent for themselves, unless the research is designed to benefit the child or children as a class. This concern was documented by Coffey, Wilfond, and Ross in a review of clinical asthma trials published before the NIH policy went into effect. They found that of fifty-two published clinical asthma trials that enrolled both children and adults, only one included a subpopulation analysis of adverse effects according to age despite the fact that some studies enrolled a significant number of children.[54] Although one may be able to extrapolate efficacy in asthma from adults to children,[55] a subgroup analysis may be useful to explore for example, possible variation in the effect size or new pediatric safety signals. Otherwise children may be exposed to the risks of research absent any compensatory scientific benefit.

Even research that only enrolls children may not provide data about children at different ages and stages of development. Contopoulos-Ioannidis and colleagues found that most studies and meta-analyses did not provide a rationale for the selection of the particular age-subgroups that they used. They concluded, "We observed large variability in the age ranges of children considered appropriate by different research teams to be included in recent pediatric trials and pediatric meta-analyses, even for trials targeting similar interventions and similar conditions" (p. 8171).[56] This also raises the justice concern of exposing children to research risks when the data cannot be extrapolated to benefit children as a class.

Looking Ahead

Experience teaches us that children are more physiologically and developmentally dynamic than adults. They are also not a monolithic group, but are a heterogeneous population. Children include premature infants, full-term infants, preschool children, school-aged children, and adolescents. Some are healthy, some are at risk, and others have a disorder or condition. Children at different ages of development activate different enzymatic pathways and metabolize chemicals differently. They clearly experience different health problems. As with adults, children come in all races and ethnicities, and live in different social and environmental conditions in all parts of the globe. We must include a diverse group of children to ensure that research addresses both the biologic and social determinants of health, and that the results are generalizable.

What, then, does justice demand in pediatric research? At minimum, justice demands an equitable balance between access to and protection from research that maximizes benefits to children as a class while minimizing harms to individual children. Justice also requires that we promote a fair selection of subjects so that we do not exploit one group (e.g., the institutionalized) to benefit the wider community and that we do not exclude one group (e.g., neonates), particularly if the disease manifests in infancy. The research must be designed to enroll sufficient numbers of children to make scientifically sound subset analyses feasible and not to enroll children merely to achieve accrual goals.

Justice also supports moving beyond the traditional medical model focused on disease and pharmaceutical treatment to a more holistic biopsychosocial model for pediatric research. In the past decade we have learned the importance of the social determinants of health. Obesity, violence, and poverty are three of the major causes of health issues that plague our children, particularly minorities and those of lower socioeconomic status. We must address these issues because they are root causes for pediatric health disparities. We have also learned in the past decade how most adult health problems originate in childhood. Thus, researchers, governments, and policymakers all need to focus resources and research on understanding the conditions under which children reach optimal health and developmental outcomes in order to reduce health disparities across the lifespan.[57,58]

Acknowledgment

This work represents the opinions of the authors and does not represent Johnson & Johnson policy.

Notes

1. Blumer J. Off-label uses of drugs in children. *Pediatrics*. 1999;104(3)(suppl 2):598–602.
2. Yoon EY, Davis MM, El-Essawi H, Cabana MD. FDA labeling status of pediatric medications. *Clinical Pediatrics*. 2006;45(1):75–77.

3. Sachs AN, Avant D, Lee CS, Rodriguz W, Murphy MD. Pediatric information in drug product labeling. *JAMA*. 2012;307(18):1914–1915.

4. Kimland E, Odlind V. Off-label drug use in pediatric patients. *Clinical Pharmacology & Therapeutics*. 2012;91(5):796–801.

5. Bellis JR, Kirkham JJ, Thiesen S, et al. Adverse drug reactions and off-label and unlicensed medicines in children: a nested case-control study of inpatients in a pediatric hospital. *BMC Medicine*. 2013;11:238.

6. Cohen E, Shaul RZ. Beyond the therapeutic orphan: children and clinical trials. *Pediatric Health*. 2008;2(2):151–159

7. Macrae D. Conducting clinical trials in pediatrics. *Critical Care Medicine*. 2009;37(1)(suppl):s136–s139.

8. Lederer SE, Grodin MA. Historical overview: pediatric experimentation. In: Grodin MA, Glantz LH, eds. *Children as Research Subjects: Science Ethics and Law*. New York, NY: Oxford University Press; 1994:3–25.

9. Beecher HK. Ethics and clinical research. *New England Journal of Medicine*. 1966;274(24):1354–1360.

10. Advisory Committee on Human Radiation Experiments. *The Human Radiation Experiments: Final Report of the President's Advisory Committee*. New York, NY: Oxford University Press; 1996.

11. Krugman S. The Willowbrook hepatitis studies revisited: ethical aspects. *Reviews of Infectious Diseases*. 1986;8(1):157–162.

12. Ramsey P. *The Patient as Person: Explorations in Medical Ethics*. New Haven, CT: Yale University Press; 1970.

13. Rothman DJ. Were Tuskegee & Willowbrook "studies in nature"? *Hastings Center Report*. 1982;12(2):5–7.

14. Kipnis K. Seven vulnerabilities in the pediatric research subject. *Theoretical Medicine and Bioethics*. 2003;24(2):107–120.

15. US Food and Drug Administration. A history of the FDA and drug regulation in the United States, 1906–2006. http://www.fda.gov/downloads/Drugs/ResourcesForYou/Consumers/BuyingUsingMedicineSafely/UnderstandingOver-the-CounterMedicines/ucm093550.pdf. Accessed November 21, 2017.

16. US Food and Drug Administration. Science and the regulation of biological products: from a rich history to a challenging future. http://www.fda.gov/AboutFDA/WhatWeDo/History/ProductRegulation/100YearsofBiologicsRegulation/ucm070022.htm. Accessed November 21, 2017.

17. Drug Efficacy Amendment of 1962. Pub L No 87–781, 76 Stat 780.

18. Chesney RW, Christensen ML. Changing requirements for evaluation of pharmacologic agents. *Pediatrics*. 2004;113(4)(suppl 3):1128–1132.

19. Shirkey H. Editorial comment: therapeutic orphans. *Journal of Pediatrics*. 1968;72(1):119–120.

20. National Research Act of 1974. Pub L No 93–348, 88 Stat 342.

21. National Commission for the Protection of Human Subjects of Biomedical and Behavioral Research. The Belmont Report: Ethical principles and guidelines for the protection of human subjects of research. *Federal Register*. 1979;44(76):23192–23197.

22. National Commission for the Protection of Human Subjects of Biomedical and Behavioral Research. *Report and Recommendations: Research Involving Children*. Washington, DC: US Government Printing Office; 1977. https://repository.library.georgetown.edu/bitstream/handle/10822/559373/Research_involving_children.pdf?sequence=1&isAllowed=y. Accessed November 21, 2017.

23. US Department of Health and Human Services. Protection of human subjects. 45 CFR 46. http://www.hhs.gov/ohrp/regulations-and-policy/regulations/45-cfr-46/. Accessed November 21, 2017.

24. US Food and Drug Administration. Protection of human subjects. 21 CFR 50. https://www.accessdata.fda.gov/scripts/cdrh/cfdocs/cfcfr/CFRSearch.cfm?CFRPart=50. Accessed November 21, 2017.

25. Field MJ, Behrman RE, eds. *Ethical Conduct of Clinical Research Involving Children*. Washington, DC: National Academies Press; 2004.

26. National Human Research Protections Advisory Committee. Children's Workgroup report from April 2001 meeting. http://wayback.archive-it.org/4657/20150930184138/http://www.hhs.gov/ohrp/archive/nhrpac/mtg04-01/child-workgroup4-5-01.pdf. Accessed November 21, 2017.

27. Secretary's Advisory Committee for Human Research Protections. Presentations and reports from April 18-19, 2005 meeting. https://wayback.archive-it.org/4657/20150930183822/http://www.hhs.gov/ohrp/archive/sachrp/mtgings/mtg04-05/present.htm. Accessed November 21, 2017.

28. Shah S, Whittle A, Wilfond B, Gensler G, Wendler D. How do institutional review boards apply the federal risk and benefit standards for pediatric research? *JAMA*. 2004;291(4):476–482.

29. Ackerman TF. Moral duties of investigators toward sick children. *IRB: A Review of Human Subjects Research*. 1981;3(6):1–5.

30. Ackerman TF. Moral duties of parents and nontherapeutic clinical research procedures involving children. *Bioethics Quarterly*. 1980;2(2):94–111.

31. Ross LF. *Children, Families and Health Care Decision-Making*. Oxford, England: Oxford University Press; 1998.

32. Bartholome WG. Parents, children, and the moral benefits of research. *Hastings Center Report*. 1976;6(6):44–45.

33. National Commission for the Protection of Human Subjects of Biomedical and Behavioral Research (NCPHS). Transcript of March 11, 1977 NCPHS meeting in Bethesda, MD. Available at the Bioethics Research Library, Georgetown University, Washington, DC.

34. Nelson RM, Ross LF. In defense of a single standard of research risk for all children. *Journal of Pediatrics*. 2005;147(5):565–566.

35. Rawls J. *A Theory of Justice*. Cambridge, MA: Harvard University Press; 1971.

36. US Department of Health and Human Services. Additional protections for children involved as subjects in research. *Federal Register*. 1983;48(46):9814–9820.

37. American Academy of Pediatrics Committee on Drugs. Guidelines for the ethical conduct of studies to evaluate drugs in pediatric populations. *Pediatrics*. 1995;95(2):286–294.

38. US Food and Drug Administration. Specific requirements on content and format of labeling for human prescription drugs; revision of "pediatric use" subsection in the labeling, Part II. *Federal Register*. 1994;59(238):64240–64250.

39. US Food and Drug Administration. Regulations requiring manufacturers to assess the safety and effectiveness of new drugs and biological products in pediatric patients. *Federal Register*. 1998;63(231):66632–66672.

40. Li JS, Eisenstein EL, Grabowski HG, et al. Economic return of clinical trials performed under the pediatric exclusivity program. *JAMA*. 2007;297(5):480–488.

41. Thaul S. *FDA's Authority to Ensure That Drugs Prescribed to Children Are Safe and Effective*. Washington, DC: Congressional Research Service; 2012. http://www.fas.org/sgp/crs/misc/RL33986.pdf. Accessed November 21, 2017.

42. Food and Drug Administration Safety and Innovation Act of 2012, Pub L No 112–114, 126 Stat 993.

43. Food and Drug Administration Reauthorization Act of 2017. Pub L No 115-52. https://www.congress.gov/bill/115th-congress/house-bill/2430/text. Accessed November 27, 2017.

44. Milne C-P, Bruss JB. The economics of pediatric formulation development for off-patent drugs. *Clinical Therapeutics*. 2008;30(11):2133–2145.

45. Pediatric Research Equity Act of 2003. Pub L No. 108-155, 117 Stat 1936.

46. National Institutes of Health. NIH policy and guidelines on the inclusion of children as participants in research involving human subjects. http://grants.nih.gov/grants/guide/notice-files/not98-024.html. Published March 6, 2008. Updated October 13, 2015. Accessed November 21, 2017.

47. New pediatric labeling information database. US Food and Drug Administration website. Pediatric Labeling Changes as of September 30, 2017. http://www.accessdata.fda.gov/scripts/sda/sdNavigation.cfm?sd=labelingdatabase. Accessed November 27, 2017.

48. US Food and Drug Administration. Pediatric exclusivity granted. http://www.fda.gov/downloads/Drugs/DevelopmentApprovalProcess/DevelopmentResources/UCM223058.pdf. Published April 2016. Accessed November 21, 2017.

49. Yang CP, Veltri MA, Anton B, Yaster M, Berkowitz ID. Food and Drug Administration approval for medications used in the pediatric intensive care unit: a continuing conundrum. *Pediatric Critical Care Medicine*. 2011;12(5):e195–e199.

50. Laughon MM, Benjamin DK Jr, Capparelli EV, et al. Innovative clinical trial design for pediatric therapeutics. *Expert Review in Clinical Pharmacology.* 2011;4(5):643–652.

51. Field MJ, Boat TF, eds. *Safe and Effective Medicines for Children.* Washington, DC: National Academies Press; 2012.

52. Kesselheim AS. An empirical review of major legislation affecting drug development: past experiences, effects, and unintended consequences. *Milbank Quarterly.* 2011;89(3):450–502.

53. Pasquali SK, Lam WK, Chiswell K, Kemper AR, Li JS. Status of the pediatric clinical trials enterprise: an analysis of the US ClinicalTrials.gov registry. *Pediatrics.* 2012;130(5):e1269–e1277.

54. Coffey MJ, Wilfond B, Ross LF. Ethical assessment of clinical asthma trials including children subjects. *Pediatrics.* 2004;113(1, pt 1):87–94.

55. Dunne J, Rodriguez WJ, Murphy MD, et al. Extrapolation of adult data and other data in pediatric drug-development programs. *Pediatrics.* 2011;128(5):e1242–e1249.

56. Contopoulos-Ioannidis DG, Seto I, Hamm MP, et al. Empirical evaluation of age groups and age-subgroup analyses in pediatric randomized trials and pediatric meta-analyses. *Pediatrics.* 2012;129(suppl 3):s161–s184.

57. Magggi S, Irwin LJ, Siddiqi A, Hertzman C. The social determinants of early child development: an overview. *Journal of Paediatrics and Child Health.* 2010;46(11):627–635.

58. Braveman PA, Egerter SA, Mockenhaupt RE. Broadening the focus: the need to address the social determinants of health. *American Journal of Preventive Medicine.* 2011;40(1)(suppl 1):s4–s18.

6 JUSTICE AND WOMEN'S PARTICIPATION IN RESEARCH

Nancy Kass
Anne Drapkin Lyerly

It is curious that the inclusion of women in biomedical research has become a justice issue. Women are different from other subpopulations addressed in this volume: unlike minority populations, women comprise 51 percent of the population; unlike children and persons with mental disabilities, women are usually competent adults; and unlike prisoners, women have no objective constraints on their autonomy. Yet over the last two decades, the issue has garnered increased attention: expert panels have been convened,[1,2] scholars have argued for greater inclusion,[3-7] data have been collected on the extent to which women and their interests have been included in clinical research,[8-10] and federal policy has become more inclusive of women.[11]

This chapter will discuss how conceptions of justice in research apply to women, why they are important, and harms that can ensue if justice is not served. After presenting data regarding women's inclusion in research, the chapter describes three research areas (cardiovascular disease, HIV disease, and pregnancy) that have not been adequately inclusive of women; examines how federal regulations have reflected and partially mitigated gender inequality in research; and discusses other factors that have contributed to differential treatment of men and women by the research establishment. Finally, the chapter will propose areas for further work to ensure gender justice in research.

Among the many conceptions of justice, at least three are relevant to justice in research for women. Distributive justice requires that the benefits and burdens of research participation be equitably distributed. Defining equity in research is more complex than ensuring that the proportion of women in studies reflects the proportion of women in the population. It requires that health problems prevalent only in women or in men are given comparable attention, and when health problems affect women and men, that analyses are conducted to examine gender differences in disease mechanisms or drug effects. Further, justice requires that the health conditions of diverse women are addressed.

Some feminist theorists argue that the distributive paradigm fails to capture an important concern of justice, namely oppression. Iris Marion Young's conception of justice[12,13] requires us to look not only at whether women have been represented in research, but also at how the nature of such representation—including how the research agenda may reinforce norms in which women and their interests are not appropriately respected. Focusing attention on the impact of medical treatment during pregnancy on fetuses and future children, without regard for its impact on the health of women themselves,[14-16] may reinforce the tendency to view women as "vessels and vectors" rather than patients in their own right. Such attention could propagate laws and policies that fail to recognize the basic rights of women when pregnant.[17]

Third, there is a role for compensatory justice. To the extent that research participation has not been equitable, there is a need to right past wrongs and give disproportionate attention to women's health needs. This will remain true until the knowledge available to guide clinical care with men and women is equitable.

Justice Over Time

Discerning whether inequities have occurred and harms have ensued is challenging. Following revelations of research abuses in the 1960s and 1970s, the focus was on the potential harms of being included in research. This "protectionist" approach led to women often being excluded from participation because of concerns about harm to potential fetuses, future children, or women themselves. Over time, justice has increasingly attended to the potential harms of being excluded from research.

Excluding women from biomedical research may harm them individually and as a group. Individual benefits of participation could include access to a therapeutic intervention, or indirect benefits such as closer monitoring,[18] free medication, or expensive testing.[19] Participation may allow access to new drugs or vaccines that hold the prospect of benefit. Women as a group may also be harmed by exclusion when women's medical needs cannot be addressed appropriately in clinical care. While men and women experience many similar health problems, there are relevant differences in how diseases manifest and in how men and women respond to treatment. Sex differences in the incidence, prevalence, symptoms, age of onset, and severity of many diseases have been documented, including rheumatoid arthritis, lupus, multiple sclerosis, major depressive disorder, schizophrenia, autism, asthma, cancer, and others.[20] Studies have documented sex differences in drug metabolism[21] and treatment response, including different rates of toxicities.[22] Such differences can be traced to differences in genetics, physiology, and environmental and experiential factors.[23]

Underrepresentation of women in clinical trials has limited the ability to study differences in drug or device response by gender. Yet drug dosing based on the "average male" without sex-specific labeling[24] can lead to "sex-dependent toxicity."[21] A 2001 report of the US General Accounting Office (GAO), a nonpartisan government agency that provides monitoring and auditing services to Congress, revealed that eight of the last ten drugs withdrawn from the market caused more adverse effects in women than men. The report concluded that the US "FDA [Food and Drug Administration] has not effectively overseen the presentation and analysis of data related to sex differences in drug development" (p. 4).[25] A 2006 study found that only 13 percent of randomized controlled trials in high-impact journals reported by sex or included sex as a covariate in modeling.[26]

Historically, incomplete information about clinical studies or their results made it difficult to determine who enrolled.[27,28] The 1997 US Food and Drug Administration Modernization Act (FDAMA) mandated registries of clinical trials information conducted under investigational new drug (IND) applications. A 2007 amendment required more types of trials to be registered and additional information submitted, including age and gender of study participants. Such information is available on ClinicalTrials.gov.[29] Yet serious information gaps remain because regulations do not require or collect enough information to discern whether or not gender gaps exist. Further, investigators do not always provide information, even when it is requested.[30] Additionally, the terminology used by bioethicists, policymakers, researchers, and the public to describe equitable inclusion varies, so determining what "fair distribution" means—or whether it has occurred—remains difficult.

More recently, reports have called attention to gender disparities that begin earlier in the research chain: studies in cell and animal research have routinely excluded female animals and failed to conduct sex-based analysis. A 2011 study[31] found male bias in animal studies in eight of ten disciplines, most prominently in neuroscience, in which single-sex studies of male animals outnumber those of females 5.5 to 1. In 2014, National Institutes of Health (NIH) director Francis Collins weighed in, noting that reliance on male models "obscures key sex differences that could guide clinical studies" (p. 282) and announced forthcoming NIH policies that will require researchers applying for grants to balance male and female cells or animals in preclinical studies absent "rigorously defined exceptions" (p. 283).[32]

Three Cases

How has research injustice harmed women's interests? Though there is disagreement regarding the extent to which women have been underrepresented in research,[7,20,33] three clinical examples bring the issues into sharper relief.

Cardiovascular disease, HIV disease, and pregnancy illustrate how justice has been interpreted and applied with regard to women, the harms that have ensued, and the impact of public policy and increased attention to gender disparities over time. These examples represent areas in which previous policies and norms allowed research to be marked by gender inequities; yet they also demonstrate areas of substantial, modest, or minimal progress over the decades during which equitable inclusion has been more broadly recognized as ethically required.

Cardiovascular Disease

Cardiovascular disease (including heart disease and stroke) has been the leading cause of mortality in US women since 1989; since 1984, the nonage adjusted number of deaths of women from cardiovascular disease have exceeded the number among men.[2] Yet before the early 1990s, large cardiovascular trials of risk factors or interventions were often conducted exclusively or predominantly with men,[3] with particular exclusion of childbearing and older women.[34–37]

A 2000 study evaluated the degree to which policy changes increased enrollment of women in cardiovascular trials, finding they were "moderately successful," but found no change in the cohorts in most smaller cardiovascular trials.[38] A 2008 review of randomized cardiovascular trials funded by the National Heart, Lung, and Blood Institute found that women represented only 27 percent of trial participants though women constitute 53 percent of patients with cardiovascular disease.[39]

Women have been harmed in several ways by underrepresentation in cardiovascular research. First, there may be insufficient information to make clinical recommendations for women regarding treatment.[40,41] Second, it may reinforce societal factors associated with disparities in cardiovascular outcomes, including treatment delays,[42] less medication,[43] and less aggressive management of chest pain for women.[44,45] While women's awareness that heart disease is the number one killer of women has increased over the last decade,[46] disparities continue due in part to clinicians' underestimation of its risk.[47] Third, simple extrapolation of research with men to recommendations for women can be inappropriate. Recent large trials suggest that aspirin be routinely recommended for the primary prevention of heart attacks in men but not in women.[48]

The study of cardiovascular disease in women has improved, however. One key example was the creation in 1991 of the Women's Health Initiative, a longitudinal study of "the major causes of death, disability, and frailty among middle aged and older women, including cardiovascular disease, cancer, and osteoporosis" (p. 275).[48] The study found a higher incidence of heart disease, stroke, and venous thromboembolism among women taking estrogen and an increased risk of stroke and venous thromboembolism among women taking estrogen and progesterone compared to women taking a placebo. These results were surprising, as cardiovascular risk reduction had been a major argument for widespread prescription of postmenopausal hormone therapy. The absence of rigorous research on hormone therapy likely put women in harm's way, and its eventual conduct, according to physician Susan Love and others, "saved many lives" (p. WK1).[49] The age-adjusted death rate from coronary heart disease is now a third of what it was in 1980, attributed in part to evidence-based improvements in cardiovascular disease prevention in women in the last decade.[50]

Nevertheless, disparities remain. A 2010 US Institute of Medicine (IOM, now known as the National Academy of Medicine) report cites an enduring lack of knowledge about sex differences in cardiovascular disease due to a lack of sex-specific analyses in studies and underenrollment of women in cardiovascular trials. Furthermore, knowledge is needed on disparities across subgroups of women, including reasons for higher coronary mortality in black compared to white women.[2]

HIV Disease

HIV disease also illustrates gender inequity in research, partially mitigated over time. A 1994 IOM panel[1] and others[15] concluded that women were underrepresented in clinical and epidemiologic HIV research, particularly in the early years of the epidemic. In 1987, federally funded epidemiologic studies of HIV targeted women primarily when the research concerned transmission through pregnancy or sex work. By 1991, ten years after the first cases of AIDS in men and in women had been reported to the US Centers for Disease Control and Prevention (CDC), there still were no large studies of HIV infection in women, despite $80 million spent on a single study of the natural history of HIV in men who have sex with men.[15] In 1993 the CDC began a study of the natural history of HIV in women; in 1994 women were enrolled in a similar NIH study.

The potential harms to women of such inequities were documented extensively.[15,51–52] Foremost was the lack of awareness on the part of medical professionals—particularly early in the epidemic—of the uniquely female manifestations of HIV; innumerable HIV–infected women who sought health care went undiagnosed and untreated. Further, the lack of systematic data documenting how HIV disease affected women prevented inclusion of female-specific manifestations of HIV, such as cervical cancer, in the CDC AIDS case definition until 1993.[53] Since social service benefits were often based on a diagnosis of AIDS as defined by the CDC,[54,55] many women living with HIV were denied public benefits that men with HIV received.

The last twenty years have seen major advances in the treatment of HIV disease. Many trials have focused on men, although reductions in morbidity and mortality have benefited women as well. A 2012 meta-analysis of randomized trials of antiretroviral treatment (ART) indicated that women represented approximately 20 percent of research participants from 2000 to 2008, although their representation has decreased since 2005.[56] Analyses indicated that ARTs were equally efficacious in men and women, though such analyses left open the possibility of undetected gender differences.[56]

Despite advances in HIV research, women's underrepresentation in HIV trials has had negative implications. Available data led the 2010 IOM Committee to conclude treatment toxicities may be more severe among women, potentially because of pharmacokinetic differences.[2] Women account for a growing proportion of individuals with HIV worldwide. In the United States, the proportion of patients with HIV disease increased from 7 percent in 1985 to 27 percent in 2007,[57] the vast majority of whom are women of color, emphasizing the importance of prevention research. Finally, in promising new areas such as "HIV Cure" research, exclusion of women of childbearing potential due to risk of reproductive toxicity has provoked significant controversy; commentators have emphasized the importance of including women in such trials.[58] Dialogue about what constitutes justification for gender-based exclusion from research will be critical to the ethical conduct of future studies.

Pregnancy

If progress has been made in many areas, there is one population that remains profoundly, and unjustly, understudied: pregnant women. Despite the 1994 IOM report's recommendation that pregnant women be "presumed to be eligible for participation in clinical studies" (p. 17), many researchers and oversight bodies continue to consider pregnancy a near automatic cause for exclusion, regardless of the harms of exclusion or the magnitude of risks of their participation. A 2013 study indicated that of all Phase IV interventional studies sponsored by the pharmaceutical industry evaluating conditions that may be experienced but are not exclusive to pregnant women, and involving a medication not classified as potentially teratogenic, only 1 percent were designed specifically for pregnant women and only 5 percent allowed pregnant women to be included.[59]

The costs of such exclusions are significant. Of the more than two hundred million women who become pregnant each year worldwide, several million experience medical illnesses. Diabetes, hypertension, psychiatric illness—even cancer—complicate hundreds of thousands of pregnancies in the United States alone;[6] malaria affects 30 million women in Africa and may account for as many as 25 percent of maternal deaths where it is endemic.[60] But evidence to guide treatment for these and other diseases in pregnancy is lacking. Few drugs are approved by the FDA for use in pregnancy: only two medications were approved specifically for use in pregnancy between 1962 and 2010.[61] All approved medications for use in pregnancy have been directed at gestation- or birth-related issues such as preterm labor prevention or regional anesthesia; any drug used to treat an underlying illness (such as diabetes or hypertension) while a woman is pregnant is prescribed during pregnancy "off label." Not until 2013 did the FDA approve a drug for treatment of morning sickness though it is the most common illness in pregnancy.[62]

Understanding how drugs work during pregnancy is important since pregnancy extends and alters the impact of sex differences on the absorption, distribution, metabolism, and excretion of drugs. Lack of evidence to guide treatment decisions results in errors in both guidelines and dosing. For instance, in the 2008 influenza epidemic, public health officials recommended that women exposed to influenza be treated with antiviral therapy at standard doses. A 2011 study, however, indicated that higher doses might be necessary to achieve therapeutic levels in pregnancy, which may partially explain the excess morbidity and mortality seen among pregnant women who contracted epidemic flu.[63]

Exclusion is further problematic in three ways. First is fetal safety: nearly 90 percent of women take medications at some point in pregnancy and approximately 50 percent take at least one prescription medication.[64] Yet the impact of such medications on fetal health is largely unknown. The teratogenic risk is unknown for 98 percent of the drugs approved between 2000 and 2010 and for nearly 90 percent of drugs approved between 1980 and 2000.[65] Without data, women and physicians cannot know which medication will be the safest choice. Second, evidence gaps have led to a reticence to use medications during pregnancy, even when harm related to untreated disease outweighs any potential toxic or teratogenic risk. For instance, untreated asthma is associated with preeclampsia, premature delivery, hemorrhage, and low birth weight, while women adequately treated have birth outcomes similar to women without asthma.[66] Third, excluding pregnant women from research harms them by denying potential benefits of research participation. For example, enhanced monitoring inherent to research may confer a safety benefit for research participation over standard clinical care.[67]

Other Factors

Several other factors play an important relationship to justice and research with women. These include federal research policies, culture, legal liability, leadership in medicine and research, and gaps in the research agenda. Each of these will be discussed in turn.

Federal Research Policies on the Inclusion of Women in Research

Federal policies have reflected and perpetuated the attitude that women of childbearing potential and pregnant women should not be enrolled in clinical research. Policies have changed over the last two decades to become more inclusive, though such policies have not gone far enough to address the remaining cultural, legal, and practical barriers to equitable inclusion of women.

Research funded by the NIH is subject to the general human subjects regulations as well as guidelines regarding inclusion of women. In response to a 1986 report of the US Public Health Service Task Force finding that, "The historical lack of research focus on women's health concerns has compromised the quality of health information available to women as well as the health care they receive,"[68] the NIH issued its first guidelines addressing gender in research, which encouraged applicants for extramural funding to include women in their studies and to offer justification if women were not included. However, in 1991 the GAO, issued a report indicating that applicants and reviewers were not aware of the NIH guidelines, there was little institutional enforcement, and there was no policy addressing the inclusion of women in intramural NIH research.[69]

In 1990, the NIH created the Office of Research on Women's Health (ORWH) "to ensure that research conducted and supported by NIH adequately addresses issues regarding women's health" (p. 44).[1] Accompanying guidelines required participation of both men and women in all extramural research and required monitoring of investigators' compliance through an-nual reports to the NIH.

Further strengthening these requirements, the creation of the ORWH was legislatively mandated through the NIH Revitalization Act of 1993 to be a focal point for women's health research at the NIH. Congress also required specific provisions in NIH guidelines for the inclusion of women and minorities in NIH–funded research.[70] This act also required that the director of NIH en-sure that "women are included as subjects in each project of such research"; that guidelines determine "the circumstances under which the inclusion of women . . . is inappropriate";[70] that Phase III trials be designed to allow valid subanalyses of intervention effect by gender and minority subgroups; and that cost not be a reason for noncompliance.[70]

The GAO issued a series of reports on the theme of inclusion of women and minorities in research and found that, as of 2000, while women were represented in NIH–funded clinical research studies at rates proportional to their numbers in the general population, "NIH has made less progress on implementing the requirement that certain clinical trials be designed and carried out to permit valid analysis by sex, which could reveal whether interventions affect men and women differently" (p. 4).[9]

Several policies regarding inclusion of women have been issued by the FDA. Regulations issued in 1977 excluded women of childbearing potential from Phase I and early Phase II trials, reflecting a concern that all drugs could be teratogenic. Even women on oral or injectable contraceptives or whose partners had had vasectomies were excluded.[1] If reproductive studies were conducted with animals (occurring less than half the time), then women of childbearing potential could, with contraceptive counseling and pregnancy testing, enroll in later Phase II and Phase III testing. Exceptions were made when the investigational drug might be lifesaving.

Revised FDA guidelines in 1988 aimed to increase scientific knowledge re-lated to women and called for assessments in dose-response by gender when women were enrolled.[71] Evaluation of these guidelines indicated that fewer than half of the new drug applications provided such subanalyses.[72] In 1993 the FDA lifted the earlier ban on enrollment of women of childbearing potential in early-phase research, acknowledged that women can modify their own be-havior to reduce fetal exposure (i.e., can be trusted to use contraceptives), and concluded that decisions about maternal and fetal risk are best left to "patients, local IRBs, and sponsors, with appropriate review and guidance by FDA."[73] It informed investigators that they are expected, although not mandated, to in-clude women in their trials and conduct subanalyses by gender. In 2000, the FDA amended its guidelines governing new drug applications, allowing the agency to discontinue a clinical trial if the sponsor proposes to exclude women based on reproductive potential. According to the FDA, their "primary intent [was] to ensure that women or men who have a life-threatening disease are not automatically excluded from investigational trials . . . due to a perceived or potential risk of developmental toxicity."[74] In 2012, the FDA published new guidance offering several strategies to improve recruitment of women and minorities into clinical trials.[75]

Federal Policies Specific to Pregnant Women

Federal policies also address research with pregnant women. Subpart B of the Department of Health and Human Services (HHS) regulations governing federally funded research states that pregnant women may be included in such a study only if ten conditions are met, including "the risk to the fetus is caused solely by interventions . . . that hold out the prospect of direct benefit for the woman or the fetus; or . . . the risk to the fetus is not greater than minimal risk."[73] Subpart B also requires the consent of both the mother and father (unless he is unavailable or the pregnancy resulted from rape or incest) for studies that hold the prospect of benefit only to the fetus.

A 1994 IOM panel recommended that Subpart B be changed to require that investigators justify exclusion rather than only inclusion of pregnant women and that pregnant women be excluded only when "an IRB finds and records its findings in writing that . . . there is no prospect of medical benefit to the pregnant woman and a risk of significant harm to potential offspring is known or can be plausibly inferred" (p. 18).[1] Further changes were suggested[76] to mandate trials on medical conditions that coexist with pregnancy, but these have not been incorporated into Subpart B. Revisions in 2001 marked a shift in language, from "no pregnant woman may be a research subject . . . unless," to "pregnant women. . . may be involved in research if," ten conditions are met; exempted from the regulations six categories of research; and provided a mechanism for the secretary of HHS to conduct or fund research not otherwise approvable after consultation with an expert panel and after public review and comment.[77] Recent changes to the federal regulations[78] did not include changes to Subpart B. However, the revised regulations no longer include pregnant women in the list of populations considered "vulnerable," which may help redress the problematic view that pregnant women should be protected from research rather than through it. In another positive move, 2017 saw the establishment of a Task Force on Research Specific to Pregnant and Lactating Women (PRGLAC) to advise the Secretary of Health and Human Services on research aimed at improving the evidence base for treatment of pregnant and lactating women.[79]

While the FDA in 1993 lifted the ban on the inclusion of women of childbearing potential in drug trials, the policy for pregnant women was unchanged.[80] In 2010, the FDA suggested that pregnant women need not always be excluded from trials, and indicated that pregnant women "may be included after all female reproduction toxicity studies and the standard battery of genotoxicity tests" are completed and safety data from previous human exposure [has been] evaluated." The FDA has indicated it is preparing draft guidance for industry on pregnant women in clinical trials."[81]

Culture

An important but hidden challenge to gender justice in research is androcentrism, the tendency to view man as the tacit standard for the "paradigmatic human."[82] As such, "normal" human functioning is generally defined as what is "normal" for men; thus, women's hormonal fluctuations are said to "complicate" research findings when they might be seen as the reason research with women is necessary to guide their treatment. As Margaret Olivia Little has argued, "Trust in all-male studies seems to reflect a broad confidence in the neutrality of treating the male body as the human norm and a familiar tendency to regard that which is distinct to woman as a distortion . . . something that is best ignored, rather than an important factor in its own right, one influencing the actual effect of the object studied" (p. 8).[83]

A second effect of androcentrism is the tendency to view women primarily in terms of their reproductive capacities. Women's health has tended to be "subsumed under obstetrics and gynecology or addressed through maternal and child health programs" (p. 5).[84] Not surprisingly, contraceptive technology for women is far more advanced than contraceptive technology for men.

Another cultural challenge to gender justice in research is distortions in how risk is perceived in pregnancy.[85] Pregnancy can intensify the already demanding standards of moral sacrifice applied to mothers, leading to a tendency to regard any risk to the fetus as unjustified—regardless of whether risks would be greater by failing to intervene. This stance is in direct tension with the research paradigm in which risks are carefully evaluated and managed in order to garner knowledge.[6]

Liability

Research exclusion of women has often been justified from fear of legal liability. Since the thalidomide and DES disasters of the 1960s and 1970s, in which women took a medication during pregnancy that resulted in their offspring suffering serious damage, clinicians and the public became aware that medications taken during pregnancy may cause harm to the fetus.[1] Further, while approximately 3 percent of pregnancies are complicated by a major congenital anomaly,[86] even anomalies unrelated to study participation could result in legal action. Concerns about legal liability have led to hesitation by industry to enroll women of childbearing age, particularly pregnant women.[87] This remains true, despite only four cases having been decided involving fetal harm in research; in each, the plaintiffs claimed that they did not give their informed consent and did not know they were part of an experiment.[87] Legal scholars have predicted that companies' failure to detect fetotoxic effects of drugs constitute greater potential for liability than research-related injury.[1,87]

Leadership

Although as of 2004 women accounted for about half of medical students, women's advancement to leadership positions has not kept pace. In 2002 women comprised only 14 percent of tenured faculty and 12 percent of full professors in academic medicine.[88] Only five of twenty-one NIH Institutes are headed by women; and women comprise less than 20 percent of the editorial boards of the three leading medical journals in the United States.[89] The first female editor of the major women's health journal *Obstetrics and Gynecology* was only appointed in 2012.[90] Women are also underrepresented in science leadership: among the Principal Investigators of NIH Clinical and Translational Science Awards (CTSAs)—one of the largest federal research grants of its type in history—only three of the first twenty-five awarded went to women.[91] Links between women's leadership in medicine and biomedical research and progress in women's health research have long been suggested.[92] A key example is the launch of the Women's Health Initiative during the tenure of Bernadine Healy, the only woman director of the National Institutes of Health.

Subgroups of Women

As attention to justice and inclusion of women in research grows, inequities among subgroups of women remain problematic. While justice in research in terms of race is discussed elsewhere in this volume, gender justice in research will not be achieved if racial disparities among women persist. Black women have a higher mortality rate from breast cancer than white women[2] and a greater risk of dying of heart disease.[2] They are approximately fifteen times as likely to contract HIV[2] and nearly three times as likely to die in childbirth.[2] The 2010 IOM report recommended that government agencies "develop targeted initiatives to increase research on the populations of women that have the highest risks and burdens of disease," such as those who "experience social disadvantage as a result of race or ethnicity, low income, or low educational level."[2]

Justice also requires considerations of other subgroups. Women are disproportionately affected when older persons are excluded from research. Globally, women constitute 55.9 percent of those over age sixty-five and 67.7 percent of those over age eighty-five.[93] Yet older persons are often excluded from research ranging from cardiovascular disease[94] to surgery for urinary incontinence.[95] And, extrapolation of data from younger patients may be harmful for elderly populations. Eliciting input about the highest priorities of older persons themselves is important.[96]

Finally, while progress has been made in understanding the social determinants of health, recent research on epigenetics has demonstrated how the environment—physical and social—affects not only health but gene expression across the lifespan. We are just beginning to understand how "social forces"—ranging from pollution to nutrition to parenting—can become "molecularly embodied" and introduce lasting changes to health.[97–99] Attention must be directed at both the biological and social factors and their interactions, and how they contribute to disparities.

Looking Ahead

The NIH Office of Research on Women's Health exists to ensure that the NIH research portfolio as a whole is attentive to the needs of women. Although time will tell the extent to which policy changes improve women's standing in research and ultimately their health, to the extent they are effective they are to be celebrated.

While women are included in research more than ever before, certain subgroups—such as pregnant women—have seen little change. Other tasks await. First, rigorous monitoring of policy changes must continue, including attention to (1) the degree to which epidemiologic research is conducted with women to identify women's greatest health needs; (2) the clinical research portfolio to determine the degree to which women's health needs are being studied; and (3) treatment trials to see if gender effects are examined as a research question.

Externally imposed policies always will have limited effectiveness if those implementing them do not believe in their importance. Health professionals should be trained early on about gender-based medicine; they should be taught that, while many medical problems manifest themselves similarly in men and women, physiology and social context can change how even common conditions and drugs differentially affect health.

Finally, having women in leadership roles can only help to advance justice in research for women.[95] Understanding the social, cultural, and other factors that either preclude women from reaching leadership goals or lead them to decide against pursuing them[100-102] will be important to ensuring that women can achieve these positions in adequate number to make necessary changes in academic medicine and the women's health research agenda. Further, diversity among women in leadership roles is key—with regard to race, ethnicity, sexual orientation, and childbearing status, among other considerations. The greater the diversity among decision-makers, the more likely it is that the needs of all persons will be recognized and included.

Conclusion

The good news is that women are now included in research more than ever. Yet a tremendous backlog of research questions remain. While exclusionary practices are undoubtedly a reflection of broader societal inequities and not their cause, each additional example of inequity with regard to gender reinforces the seeming normalcy of such practices. By the same token, each step toward dismantling inequities has an impact beyond its own small world.

The true test will be not only in the research portfolio five or ten years from now, but also in determining the extent to which health-care providers understand women's health needs and in examining future outcomes with regard to the health status of women.

Notes

1. Mastroianni AC, Faden R, Federman D, eds. *Women and Health Research: Ethical and Legal Issues of Including Women in Clinical Studies.* Vol. 1. Washington, DC: National Academies Press; 1994.
2. Institute of Medicine. *Women's Health Research: Progress, Pitfalls and Promise.* Washington, DC: National Academies Press; 2010.
3. Dresser R. Wanted: single, white male for medical research. *Hastings Center Report.* 1992;22(1):24–29.
4. Kass NE, Taylor HA, King PA. Harms of excluding pregnant women from clinical research: the case of HIV-infected women. *Journal of Law, Medicine & Ethics.* 1996; 24(1):36–46.
5. Merton V. The exclusion of pregnant, pregnable, and once-pregnable people (a.k.a. women) from biomedical research. *American Journal of Law & Medicine.* 1993;19(4):369–451.

6. Lyerly AD, Little MO, Faden R. The second wave: toward the responsible inclusion of pregnant women in research. *International Journal of Feminist Approaches to Bioethics*. 2008; 1(2):5–22.

7. Greenberger P. Flaunting the feminine side of research studies. *Science*. 2008;322(5906):1325–1326.

8. Schmucker DL, Vesell ES. Underrepresentation of women in clinical drug trials. *Clinical Pharmacology & Therapeutics*. 1993;54(1):11–15.

9. US General Accounting Office. *Women's Health: NIH Has Increased Its Efforts to Include Women in Research*. Washington, DC: US General Accounting Office; 2000. http://www.gao.gov/archive/2000/he00096.pdf. Accessed December 9, 2017.

10. Oertelt-Prigion S, Parol R, Krohn S, Preibner R, Regitz-Zagrosek V. Analysis of sex and gender-specific research reveals a common increase in publications and marked differences between disciplines. *BMC Medicine*. 2010:8: 70.

11. National Institutes of Health. NIH policy and guidelines on the inclusion of women and minorities as subjects in clinical research–amended, October 2001. https://grants.nih.gov/grants/funding/women_min/guidelines_amended_10_2001.htm. Accessed December 9, 2017.

12. Young IM. *Justice and the Politics of Difference*. Princeton, NJ: Princeton University Press; 1990.

13. DeBruin DA. Justice and the inclusion of women in clinical studies: an argument for further reform. *Kennedy Institute of Ethics Journal*. 1994;4(2):117–146.

14. Rosenfield A, Maine D. Maternal mortality—a neglected tragedy: where is the M in MCH? Lancet. 1985;326(8446):83–85.

15. Faden R, Kass N, McGraw D. Women as vessels and vectors: lessons from the HIV epidemic. In: Wolf S, ed. *Feminism & Bioethics: Beyond Reproduction*. New York, NY: Oxford University Press; 1996:252–281.

16. Lyerly AD, Little MO, Faden RR. The National Children's Study: a golden opportunity to advance the health of pregnant women. *American Journal of Public Health*. 2009;99(10):1742–1745.

17. Paltrow LM, Flavin J. Arrests and forced interventions on pregnant women in the United States, 1973–2005: implications for women's legal status and public health. *Journal of Health Politics, Policy and Law*. 2013;38(2):299–343.

18. Lyerly AD, Little MO, Faden RR. Reframing the framework: toward fair inclusion of pregnant women as participants in research. *American Journal of Bioethics*. 2011;11(5):50–52.

19. Merton V. Ethical obstacles to the participation of women in biomedical research. In: Wolf SM, ed. *Feminism & Bioethics: Beyond Reproduction*. New York, NY: Oxford University Press; 1996:216–251.

20. Kim AM, Tingen CM, Woodruff TK. Sex bias in trials and treatment must end. *Nature*. 2010;465(10):688–689.

21. Skett P. Biochemical basis of sex differences in drug metabolism. *Pharmacology & Therapeutics*. 1988;38(3):269–304.

22. Miller MA. Gender-based differences in the toxicity of pharmaceuticals—the Food and Drug Administration's perspective. *International Journal of Toxicology.* 2001;20(3):149–152.

23. Wizemann TM, Pardue M, eds. *Exploring the Biological Contributions to Human Health: Does Sex Matter?* Washington, DC: National Academies Press; 2001.

24. Anderson GD. Sex and racial differences in pharmacological response: where is the evidence? *Journal of Women's Health.* 2005;14(1):19–29.

25. US General Accounting Office. *Women's Health: Women Sufficiently Represented in New Drug Testing, but FDA Oversight Needs Improvement.* Washington, DC: US General Accounting Office; 2001.

26. Geller SE, Adams MG, Carnes M. Adherence to federal guidelines for reporting of sex and race/ethnicity in clinical trials. *Journal of Women's Health.* 2006;15(10):1123–1131.

27. McCray AT, Ide NC. The design and implementation of a national clinical trials registry. *Journal of the American Medical Informatics Association.* 2000;7(3):313–323.

28. Zarin DA, Ide NC, Tse T, Harlan WR, West JC, Lindberg DA. Issues in the registration of clinical trials. *JAMA.* 2007;297(19):2112–2120.

29. Background. Clinicaltrials.gov website. http://clinicaltrials.gov/ct2/about-site/background. Accessed December 9, 2017.

30. Dickersin K, Rennie D. The evolution of trial registries and their use to assess the clinical trial enterprise. *JAMA.* 2012;307(17):1861–1864.

31. Beery AK, Zucker I. Sex bias in neuroscience and biomedical research. *Neuroscience & Biobehavioral Reviews.* 2011;35(3):565–572.

32. Clayton JA, Collins FS. Policy: NIH to balance sex in cell and animal studies. *Nature.* 2014;509(7500):282–283.

33. Holden C. Women abound in NIH trials. *Science.* 2008;322(5899):219.

34. Wenger NK, Speroff L, Packard B. Cardiovascular health and disease in women. *New England Journal of Medicine.* 1993;329(4):247–256.

35. Murphy ML, Hultgren HN, Detre K, Thomsen J, Takaro T. Treatment of chronic stable angina: a preliminary report of survival data of the randomized Veterans Administration Cooperative Study. *New England Journal of Medicine.* 1977;297(12):621–627.

36. Multiple Risk Factor Intervention Trial Research Group. Multiple risk factor intervention trial: risk factor changes and mortality results. *JAMA.* 1982;248(12):1465–1477.

37. Manson JE, Grobbee DE, Stampfer MJ, et al. Aspirin in the primary prevention of angina pectoris in a randomized trial of United States physicians. *American Journal of Medicine.* 1990;89(6):772–776.

38. Harris DJ, Douglas PS. Enrollment of women in cardiovascular clinical trials funded by the National Heart, Lung and Blood Institute. *New England Journal of Medicine.* 2000;343(7):475–480.

39. Kim ES, Carrigan TP, Menon V. Enrollment of women in National Heart, Lung, and Blood Institute-funded cardiovascular randomized controlled trials fails to meet current federal mandates for inclusion. *Journal of the American College of Cardiology.* 2008;52(8):672–673.

40. National Cholesterol Education Program. *Report of the Expert Panel on Detection, Evaluation and Treatment of High Blood Cholesterol in Adults.* Rockville, MD: National Institutes of Health; 1989.

41. LaRosa JC, He J, Vupputuri S. Effect of statins on risk of cardiovascular disease: a meta-analysis of randomized controlled trials. *JAMA.* 1999;282(24):2340–2346.

42. Jackson RE, Anderson W, Peacock WF, Vaught L, Carley RS, Wilson AG. Effect of a patient's sex on the timing of thrombolytic therapy. *Annals of Emergency Medicine.* 1996;27(1):8–15.

43. Herholz H, Goff DC, Ramsey DJ, et al. Women and Mexican Americans receive fewer cardiovascular drugs following myocardial infarction than men and non-Hispanic whites: the Corpus Christi Heart Project, 1988–1990. *Journal of Clinical Epidemiology.* 1996;49(3):279–287.

44. Schulman KA, Berlin JA, Harless W, et al. The effect of race and sex on physicians' recommendations for cardiac catheterization. *New England Journal of Medicine.*1999;340(8):618–626.

45. Chang AM, Mumma B, Sease KL, Robey JL, Shofer FS, Hollander JE. Gender bias in cardiovascular testing persists after adjustment for presenting character-istics and cardiac risk. *Academic Emergency Medicine.* 2007;14(7):599–605.

46. Mosca L, Mochari-Greenberger H, Dolor RJ, Newby LK, Robb KJ. Twelve-year follow-up of American women's awareness of cardiovascular disease risk and barriers to heart health. *Circulation: Cardiovascular Quality and Outcomes.* 2010;3(2):120–127.

47. Mosca L, Barrett-Connor E, Wegner NK. Sex/gender differences in cardio-vascular disease prevention: what a difference a decade makes. *Circulation.* 2011;124(19):2145–2154.

48. Healy B. The Yentl Syndrome. *New England Journal of Medicine.* 1991;325(4):274–276.

49. Parker-Pope T. The Women's Health Initiative and the body politic. *New York Times,* April 10, 2011:WK1.

50. Mosca L, Benjamin EJ, Berra K, et al. Effectiveness-based guidelines for the pre-vention of cardiovascular disease in women—2011 Update: a guideline from the American Heart Association. *Journal of the American College of Cardiology.* 2011;57(12):1404–1423.

51. Corea G. The Invisible Epidemic: *The Story of Women and AIDS.* New York, NY: Harper Collins; 1992.

52. Stoll KD. *Women and the Definition of AIDS.* Washington, DC: Center for Women Policy Studies; 1992.

53. Centers for Disease Control and Prevention. 1993 revised classification system for HIV infection and expanded surveillance case definition for AIDS among adolescents and adults. *MMWR Recommendations and Reports*. 1992;41(RR-17):1–19.

54. Levine C, Stein GL. What's in a name? The policy implications of the CDC definition of AIDS. *Journal of Law, Medicine and Health Care*. 1991;19(3–4):278–290.

55. Office of Technology Assessment. *The CDC's Case Definition of AIDS: Implications of the Proposed Revisions*. Washington, DC: US Congress; 1992. HIV-Related Issues; background paper 8.

56. Soon GG, Min M, Strumble KA, et al. Meta-analysis of gender differences in efficacy outcomes for HIV-positive subjects in randomized controlled clinical trials of antiretroviral therapy (2000–2008). *AIDS Patient Care STDS*. 2012;26(8):444–453.

57. American College of Obstetricians and Gynecologists. Practice Bulletin No.117: gynecologic care for women with Human Immunodeficiency Virus. *Obstetrics & Gynecology*. 2010;116(6):1492–1509.

58. Lo B, Grady C; Working Group on Ethics of the International AIDS Society. Ethical considerations in HIV cure research: points to consider. *Current Opinion in HIV and AIDS*. 2013;8(3):243–249.

59. Shields K, Lyerly AD. Exclusion of pregnant women from industry sponsored clinical trials. *Obstetrics & Gynecology*. 2013;122(5):1077–1081.

60. Schantz-Dunn J, Nour NM. Malaria and pregnancy: a global perspective. Reviews in Obstetrics and Gynecology. 2009;2(3):186–192.

61. Wing DA, Powers B, Hickok D. US Food and Drug Administration drug approval: slow advances in obstetric care in the United States. *Obstetrics & Gynecology*. 2010;115(4):825–833.

62. Lyerly AD, Faden RR. Mothers matter: ethics and research during pregnancy. *Virtual Mentor*. 2013;15(9):775–778.

63. Beigi RH, Han K, Venkataramanan R, et al. Pharmacokinetics of oseltamivir among pregnant and non-pregnant women. *American Journal of Obstetrics & Gynecology*. 2011;204(6):s84–s88.

64. Mitchell AA, Gilboa SM, Werler MM, et al. Medication use during pregnancy, with particular focus on prescription drugs: 1978–2008. *American Journal of Obstetrics & Gynecology*. 2011;205(1):e1–e8.

65. Adam MP, Polifka JE, Friedman JM. Evolving knowledge of teratogenicity of medications in human pregnancy. *American Journal of Medical Genetics Part C: Seminars in Medical Genetics*. 2011;157C(3):175–182.

66. Dombrowski MP. Asthma and pregnancy. *Obstetrics & Gynecology*. 2006;108(3):667–681.

67. Lyerly AD, Little MO, Faden RR. Reframing the framework: toward fair inclusion of pregnant women as participants in research. *American Journal of Bioethics*. 2011;11(5):50–52.

68. US Public Health Service. Women's Health: Report of the Public Health Service Task Force on Women's Health Issues. *Public Health Reports.* 1985;100(1):73–106.

69. Hearings before the Health and the Environment Subcommittee of the House Committee on Energy and Commerce, 101st Cong, 1st Sess (1990) (testimony of Mark V. Nadel, US General Accounting Office Associate Director).

70. NIH Revitalization Act of 1993, Pub L No. 103–43, 107 Stat 122, §492B(a)(1).

71. U.S. Food and Drug Administration. *Guideline for the Format and Content of the Clinical and Statistical Sections of the New Drug Applications.* Rockville, MD: US Department of Health and Human Services; 1988.

72. US Food and Drug Administration. Guideline for the study and evaluation of gender differences in the clinical evaluation of drugs. *Federal Register.* 1993;58(139):39406–39416.

73. US Department of Health and Human Services. Protection of human subjects: research involving pregnant women or fetuses. 45 CFR §46.204(b). http://www.hhs.gov/ohrp/regulations-and-policy/regulations/45-cfr-46/#. Revised January 15, 2009. Effective July 14, 2009. Accessed December 9, 2017.

74. US Food and Drug Administration. Clinical hold for products intended for life threatening conditions. *Federal Register.* 2000;65(106):34963–34971.

75. Society for Women's Health Research; US Food and Drug Administration Office of Women's Health. *Proceedings from Dialogues on Diversifying Clinical Trials: Successful Strategies for Engaging Women and Minorities in Clinical Trials.* Washington, DC: US Food and Drug Administration; 2011. http://www.fda.gov/downloads/ScienceResearch/SpecialTopics/WomensHealthResearch/UCM334959.pdf. Accessed December 9, 2017.

76. Kass NE, Sugarman J, Faden R, Schoch-Spana M. Trust, the fragile foundation of contemporary biomedical research. *Hastings Center Report.* 1996;26(5):25–29.

77. US Department of Health and Human Services. Protection of human research subjects. *Federal Register.* 2001;66(11):3878–3883.

78. Office for Human Research Protections. Final revisions to the Federal Policy for the Protection of Human Subjects, January 19th 2017. https://www.gpo.gov/fdsys/pkg/FR-2017-01-19/html/2017-01058.htm. Accessed November 30, 2017.

79. Task Force on Research Specific to Pregnant and Lactating Women. National Institute of Child Health and Human Development. https://www.nichd.nih.gov/about/meetings/2017/Pages/082117.aspx. Accessed December 15, 2017.

80. Macklin R. Enrolling pregnant women in biomedical research. *Lancet.* 2010;375(9715):632–633.

81. FDA's guidance document to-do list. Pink Sheet website. https://pink.pharmamedtechbi.com/PS052984/FDArsquos-Guidance-Document-ToDo-List. Accessed October 28, 2016.

82. Bem SL. The Lenses of Gender: Transforming the Debate on Sexual Inequality. New Haven, CT: Yale University Press; 1994.

83. Little MO. Why a feminist approach to bioethics? Kennedy Institute of Ethics Journal. 1996;6(1):1–18.

84. Johnson T and Fee E. Women's participation in clinical research: From protectionism to access. In: Mastroianni A, Faden R, Federman D, eds. *Women and Health Research, Ethical and Legal Issues of Including Women in Clinical Studies*, Vol. 2. Washington DC: National Academies Press, 1994.

85. Lyerly AD, Mitchell LM, Armstrong EM, et al. Risk and the pregnant body. *Hastings Center Report*. 2009;39(6):34–42.

86. Birth defects. Centers for Disease Control and Prevention website. http://www.cdc.gov/ncbddd/birthdefects/data.html. Accessed December 9, 2017.

87. Greenwood K. The mysteries of pregnancy: the role of law in solving the problem of unknown but knowable maternal-fetal medication risk. *University of Cincinnati Law Review*. 2010;79(267):267–322.

88. Bickel J, Wara D, Atkinson BF, et al. Increasing women's leadership in academic medicine: report of the AAMC Project Implementation Committee. *Academic Medicine*. 2002;77(10):1043–1061.

89. Lindemann H. The woman question in medicine: an update. *Hastings Center Report*. 2012;42(3):38–45.

90. Nancy C. Chescheir, MD, selected as the new editor-in-chief of Obstetrics & Gynecology [announcement]. *Obstetrics & Gynecology*. 2012;120(2):223.

91. Carnes M, Bland C. Viewpoint: a challenge to academic health centers and the National Institutes of Health to prevent unintended gender bias in the selection of clinical and translational science award leaders. *Academic Medicine*. 2007;82(2):202–206.

92. Carnes M, Morrisey C, Geller SE. Women's health and women's leadership in academic medicine: hitting the same glass ceiling? *Journal of Women's Health*. 2008;17(9):1453–1461.

93. International data base world population by age and sex. US Census Bureau website. http://www.census.gov/population/international/data/idb/worldpop.php. Accessed October 28, 2016.

94. Lee PY, Alexander KP, Hammill BG, Pasquali SK, Peterson ED. Representation of elderly persons and women in published randomized trials of acute coronary syndromes. *JAMA*. 2001;286(6):708–713.

95. Morse AN, Labin LC, Young SB, Aronson MP, Gurwitz JH. Exclusion of elderly women from published randomized trials of stress incontinence surgery. *Obstetrics & Gynecology*. 2004;104(3):498–593.

96. Patient-Centered Outcomes Research Institute website. http://pcori.org. Accessed December 9, 2017.

97. Landecker H, Panofsky A. From social structure to gene regulation, and back: a critical introduction to environmental epigenetics for sociology. *Annual Review of Sociology*. 2013;39(1):333–357.

98. Shulevitz J. Why fathers really matter. *New York Times*, September 9, 2012:SR1.

99. Paul AM. *Origins: How the Nine Months Before Birth Shape the Rest of Our Lives.* New York, NY: Free Press; 2010.

100. Slaughter AM. Why women still can't have it all. *The Atlantic*, July/August, 2012. http://www.theatlantic.com/magazine/archive/2012/07/why-women-still-cant-have-it-all/309020/. Accessed December 9, 2017.

101. Sandberg S. *Lean In: Women, Work, and the Will to Lead.* New York, NY: Knopf; 2013.

102. Stone P. *Opting Out: Why Women Really Quit Careers and Head Home.* Berkeley: University of California Press; 2008.

7 JUSTICE, RACE, AND RACISM IN RESEARCH

Patricia A. King

The concept of race emerged in full bloom in the eighteenth and nineteenth centuries in the United States and other countries to explain or classify observable differences among human beings. In the United States physicians and scientists used these concepts to develop much of the theory and data that supported beliefs about inherent biological differences between blacks and whites and the "inherent superiority" of whites over blacks. These beliefs defined diseases such as sickle cell anemia in racial terms, provided support for the institution of slavery, reinforced negative stereotypes about blacks and black health, and in the postemancipation era justified segregation and efforts to deny African Americans the opportunity to participate as full citizens of the country.[1*]

Understanding the African American experience in research, health care, and society is essential to ensure that justice is respected and that African Americans benefit from research advances. Toward that end, this chapter considers three research projects in which African Americans were unjustly treated. Their examination is intended to show that these injustices are less about bad intent than about reliance on biological explanations for human differences, implicit bias, stereotyping, and lack of respect for black self-determination embedded in professional practices, institutional

---

* This chapter discusses the experiences of people in the United States who trace their ancestry to African slaves. The relationship between blacks and whites has special relevance given the institution of slavery and the civil rights movement. Other racial and ethnic groups have separate and distinct experiences with American medicine and research. Although this chapter focuses on African Americans, in a broad sense the various means by which African Americans have suffered injustices in health-related contexts may be relevant to understanding how other groups in the United States and abroad are disadvantaged in research and health settings. I use the terms *black* and *African American* interchangeably.

approaches to decision-making, and the design and implementation of measures to protect research participants. This exploration underscores the need for careful attention to the hierarchies of power that take place in health-related encounters and to the contexts in which illness, treatment, and healing occur in contemporary clinical, genomic, and public health research. Such a historical and social understanding is essential to identify and address critical questions and perspectives relevant to contemporary research practices and policies.

Justice Over Time

The relationship between medicine and African Americans was shaped by slavery and the nation's political struggles before and after the Civil War. Although slavery and segregation are in the past and formal discrimination is no longer legally permitted, beliefs about white supremacy, biological explanations of differences between blacks and whites, and negative generalizations or stereotypes about the culture and behaviors of blacks as individuals or a group persist and have evolved with American culture. Given America's history, it should be no surprise to find white privilege so ingrained in institutional practices, habits of mind, and unexamined customs that few notice its presence. In the following discussion of three twentieth-century cases, these beliefs, biological explanations for difference, and negative perceptions of African Americans are uncovered. These beliefs continue to cast a long shadow.

The Tuskegee Syphilis Study

Biological understandings of racial difference in the United States promoted by scientists and medical professionals defined the relationships between medicine and African Americans in the eighteenth and nineteenth centuries. That relationship is present in the Tuskegee Syphilis Study, which is not the only example of black people being abused in a medical context but has become the epitome of such exploitation. This study sponsored by the US Public Health Service (PHS) in Macon County, Alabama, began in 1932 and involved 399 black men with syphilis and 201 controls. The study, intended solely to track the effects of untreated syphilis in black men, lasted for forty years and ended in July 1972 when Associated Press reporter Jean Heller brought the experiment to public attention.[2] The study offered no promise of benefit to the participants. The study participants were not offered the best available treatment of the time (though in retrospect it would not have been of much help in the pre-penicillin era). Moreover, the subjects were not given penicillin when it became available as an effective treatment for syphilis in the 1940s. Indeed, extensive measures were employed to keep the men from being treated. Though many of the aforementioned practices flagrantly violated what are now commonly understood to be basic ethical practices, it is the context of racism underlying the researchers' choices that can teach us the importance of integrating the perspectives of marginalized groups into current and future study designs. Lerner and Caplan ask, "Why, in the case of the Tuskegee study, did otherwise progressive persons remain so backward when it came to the issue of race? Indeed, it is precisely the context that holds the key lesson for modern researchers and clinicians studying the moral failings of their predecessors" (p. 555).[3]

Although there had been a report of a previous retrospective study of untreated syphilis in whites in Norway, PHS physicians and funders believed that it had not conclusively resolved the question of whether the course of the disease in blacks and whites might be different. Assumptions about biological differences between blacks and whites embedded in the investigators' culture undoubtedly made it difficult for them to be objective. It should be noted, however, that the historian, social critic, and activist W. E. B. DuBois writing as early as 1906 had documented disparities between whites and blacks in certain diseases and significantly raised the question whether the disparities were racial. He concluded that disparities could be explained on other grounds and that a focus on social and economic conditions would almost entirely eliminate race.[4] Nonetheless, negative stereotypes about blacks played an important role in shaping the design and implementation of the study. For example, the PHS researchers and funders believed blacks had an inherently different sexual nature than whites, blacks would not seek treatment for syphilis, and blacks were promiscuous.[5] Historian Evelyn Higginbotham notes that the decision not to treat the men in the study after penicillin became available not only demonstrated lack of concern for the men in the study, "but its even lesser concern for black women in relationships with these men. Black women failed to receive so much as a pretense of protection, so widely accepted was the belief that the spread of the disease was inevitable because black women were promiscuous by nature" (p. 265).[6] Sadly, as James Jones points out, the researchers also ignored the plight of innocent children born with the disease.[2]

In designing the study, the PHS physicians took advantage of the subjects' bleak social and economic situation in order to advance their research goals. The study took place in a rural, poor, and segregated community in the Deep South during the Great Depression. Access to basic health care and other valued amenities of life were minimal. Knowing this, the researchers offered health care services, such as free physical examinations otherwise unavailable to the participants as a way to induce participation. The PHS researchers obtained bodies for postmortem examination by promising to pay burial expenses.

The subjects did not give consent to participation. Indeed, the 1973 *Final Report* of the Tuskegee Syphilis Study Ad Hoc Advisory Panel created by the US Department of Health, Education, and Welfare (a predecessor agency to the Department of Health and Human Services) viewed the syphilis study as "ethically unjustified in 1932" because the participants had not given consent rather than because the principle of justice was violated (p. 7).[7] Social historian Allan Brandt, however, criticized the report for its focus on informed consent because it served to conceal the historical context of the study.[5] The men were denied important information not just initially but throughout the study. For example, the men thought that the lumbar punctures into the spinal cord were performed for therapeutic reasons. In fact, the punctures were used for diagnostic purposes to learn whether the men had neurosyphilis. These punctures were painful and could result in severe headaches, and in rare cases paralysis or death. Moreover, the men lived in a coercive environment. They were accustomed in the deeply segregated South to being obedient to authority, especially white authority. While all studies need subjects, these men in particular were used as means rather than respected as people with agency.

The researchers who conceived the Tuskegee Syphilis Study did not necessarily act with base motives. They may have considered themselves well-intentioned researchers focused on the pursuit of scientific knowledge, but blind to the fact that the subjects were human beings and not objects. It is even possible that at a conscious level they saw themselves as advancing the health needs of African Americans. If so, the study demonstrates how scientific objectivity can be infected with bias prevalent in the broader society. Allan Brandt has noted, "the Tuskegee Study revealed more about the pathology of racism than it did about the pathology of syphilis; more about the nature of scientific inquiry than the nature of the disease process" (p. 27).[5]

The Saga of Henrietta Lacks and Her Family

Henrietta Lacks was an African American woman born in 1920 and raised in Virginia. She was a poor farmer who, with no more than a seventh-grade education, tilled the same tobacco fields once worked by her slave forebears. At age twenty-one, she and her family joined the "Great Migration," the flood of black families moving north in search of a better life, in her case to Turner

Station near Baltimore, Maryland. There, after complications in childbirth, Lacks sought treatment at Johns Hopkins Hospital, the nearest facility willing to treat black patients, albeit in segregated facilities. She was subsequently diagnosed with cervical cancer and later died in 1951 at age thirty-one. During Henrietta Lacks's course of treatment tissue samples from her cervical cancer were collected without her permission (a common practice at the time) and given to Dr. George Gey, who worked at Johns Hopkins.[8] Gey was interested in tissue culture. He wanted to create permanent strains of human cells for experimental use in scientific research. Lacks' cancer cells were cultured in the laboratory and unlike previously collected cells from other patients, the cells did not die after several cell divisions but continued to grow and replicate. The HeLa cell line, coded according to her name, has been used extensively by scientists for more than sixty years, becoming the most plentiful and widely used human cells in medical research. The cell line is linked with significant scientific advances such as the development of the polio vaccine.

As will be revealed shortly, Henrietta Lacks's story and society's use of HeLa cells raise many ethical issues that resonate in other contexts today, among them informed consent, ownership of biological materials, and protection of individual and family privacy. Her life story further illustrates the power of negative stereotypes and the reach of the oral tradition in the African American community.

Just as Lacks and her family were linked to slavery through land and occupation, they were similarly connected to earlier attitudes and beliefs held by blacks concerning their relationship with physicians and medical institutions. African Americans emerged from slavery with strong motivation to control their own bodies in the aftermath of a collective memory of subjugation and commoditization, distrust of white health care and institutions, and, as historian Sharla Fett points out, "a storehouse of healing knowledge" (p. x).[9] Conceivably, Lacks might have turned to alternative healing knowledge. For example, Lacks's daughter Deborah utilized preaching, faith healing, and sometimes voodoo.[8] Looked at from the perspective of Western-trained physicians, this reliance on home-grown remedies might seem irresponsible or superstitious. Viewed from the perspective of those who employ alternative methods, however, it might be rational to be suspicious of the motives and practices of hospitals and conventional Western medicine. Use of alternative healing knowledge might be rationally understood as an attempt by subjugated individuals to maintain control over their bodies.

Rebecca Skloot in her book *The Immortal Life of Henrietta Lacks* notes that at least one member of the Lacks family distrusted Johns Hopkins Hospital, stating she would not go there for care because in her view the hospital had experimented on black people. She believed that "night doctors" snatched blacks from the streets and took them to hospitals for mutilation and experimentation (p. 165).[8] As Skloot points out:

> Since at least the 1800s, black oral history has been filled with tales of "night doctors" who kidnapped black people for research. . . . To discourage slaves from meeting or escaping, slave owners told tales of gruesome research done on black bodies, then covered themselves in white sheets and crept around at night posing as spirits coming to infect black people with disease or steal them for research. (pp. 165–166)[8]

Night riders in the American South have a long history of exerting psychological pressure to control blacks. Fry observes:

> Originally practiced during slavery by masters and overseers dressed as ghosts, psychological control was later extended to the system of mounted patrols (or "patterollers") designed to monitor slave movement in antebellum days, the Ku Klux Klan of the reconstruction era, and finally the night doctors. . . . [A]ll three adhered to a single cardinal purpose: the control of the Black through intimidation. (p. 3)[10]

Today in poor Baltimore neighborhoods, residents' distrust of Baltimore's medical institutions and physicians persists.[11,12]

It is possible that Lacks went to Johns Hopkins with some trepidation about more than her symptoms. In the 1950s, Henrietta Lacks's options for medical care were limited both by poverty and limited literacy, as well as by segregation in the delivery of health care. Lacks did not enjoy a personal relationship with a private doctor; consequently, there was no continuity of care for medical issues. When the need for medical care became urgent, she had no choice but to seek care in a segregated hospital in one of the few institutions that would help her. Sociologist Hannah Landecker notes that before her biopsy Lacks was initially tested for syphilis. Landecker observes that this was "a detail that should be viewed in the context of American medical history. James Jones has written about the characterization of American blacks as a notoriously syphilis-soaked race by a white medical establishment and the role of this perception in the founding of the Tuskegee syphilis experiments . . ."(p. 128).[13] This detail is suggestive of a doctor's or institution's possible bias about the patient, and serves as reminder that health care when provided was often linked with a racist view of the recipient. As historian Elizabeth Fee observes, "venereal diseases are inevitably associated with sexuality, and therefore our perceptions of these diseases tend to be entangled with our ideas about the social meanings and moral evaluation of sexual behaviors" (pp. 141–142).[14] In the case of syphilis, a physician might appreciate that the disease was caused by a specific microorganism, yet might describe the cause of the disease as promiscuous sexual behavior.

A less well-known aspect of the HeLa cells story is the way in which scientific regard for the cell line was negatively transformed in the 1960s, leading to reification of race and reinforcing stereotypes of African American women. In 1966, geneticist Dr. Stanley Gartler announced to the consternation of the cell culture community that many different human cell lines had been contaminated by HeLa cells. Gartler's evidence for his statement focused on a particular genetic enzyme, a variant that was believed to be found only in "Negroes." Gartler had previously verified that the HeLa cell line was derived from a black person. As Landecker states, "[a]fter 1966, the race of the donor was central to the scientific evidence of cell culture contamination, and metaphors and stereotypes of race framed scientific and journalistic accounts of the cell line" (p. 169).[13] The rapid reproduction of the cells, which had originally been a positive feature of the cell line, was linked negatively with metaphors about promiscuity (cells with wild proliferative tendencies), miscegenation (one drop was enough to contaminate), and reproduction out of control (cells characterized as voracious and aggressive).[15]

Ironically, the cell contamination issue, with its introduction of Lacks's race and its accompanying stereotypes, also led to the involvement of the Lacks family. Before that time the family did not know about the cell line's contributions to science. Only after the contamination scandal did the scientific community approach the family. In the 1970s, it was determined that the way to resolve the cell contamination problem was to find genetic markers specific to Henrietta Lacks and then use the markers to identify her cells and distinguish them from others. Procuring DNA samples from her husband and children identified genetic markers that were specific to Lacks. According to Skloot, the Lacks family's provision of blood samples was not accompanied by written consent, and it is unlikely that the family understood that the blood draws were not for their benefit but for the benefit of science. In Skloot's account, while the family was proud of Henrietta Lacks's contributions to science, they were also puzzled that they did not benefit from scientific commercialization of the cell line. As Ms. Lacks's daughter comments: "But I always have thought it was strange, if our mother cells done so much for medicine, how come her family can't afford to see no doctors?" (p. 9).[8] Indeed, her questioning of benefiting from the products derived from an individual's tissue is one that has been raised today by others, on both moral and legal (although to date unsuccessful) grounds.

More recently, the scientific community evidenced further disrespect of the Lacks family and their privacy interests in March 2013 when scientists in Europe published the genome of the HeLa cell line without the knowledge or consent of the Lacks family. The presumably well-meaning scientists did not break any laws. They undoubtedly saw the HeLa cell genome as an important resource for science. But they also prompted an ethics discussion about genetic privacy of family members of research subjects and the genetic privacy of the Lacks family specifically.

Fortunately, in this latest episode the US federal government intervened to work with the family to achieve a just resolution of the matter. On August 7, 2013, the family and the National Institutes of Health (NIH) announced an agreement that finally gives some recognition to the Lacks family and allows them to play a partnership role in the science that uses the HeLa cell line in the future.[16] Specifically, the agreement restricts NIH–financed research on the genome of the HeLa cells and places two family members on the HeLa Genome Data Access Working Group that approves such research.[17]

HeLa cells helped make possible important and significant advances in science. The saga of Lacks and her family, however, should remind research participants and all of those engaged in the science enterprise that making advances for the "greater good" may sometimes exploit or overlook those who lack power and are vulnerable in numerous ways. Patients and hopefully all participants in the research enterprise should appreciate that the zealous pursuit of science and the interests of professionals and institutions rather than the needs of patients or subjects in clinical research may influence decision-making in medicine and research. Finally, however, the story of the Lacks family will undoubtedly become a fixture in the collective memories of blacks, thus reinforcing a legacy of mistrust.

The Kennedy Krieger Institute's Lead Paint Study

In 2001, Maryland's highest court handed down a complex and controversial decision that resurrected consideration of ethical issues about the participation of children in a research study that was approved in the early 1990s.[18] The case, *Grimes v. Kennedy Krieger Institute, Inc.*, involved two mothers of two African American children living in low-income housing. (Although only two African American families were plaintiffs in the Grimes lawsuit, the total number of subjects in the study was 108 low-income African American households.[19]) The children had been enrolled in a study examining different partial lead abatement interventions in low-income housing units. The study was funded by the Environmental Protection Agency and conducted under the auspices of the Kennedy Krieger Institute (KKI) in Baltimore whose researchers are affiliated with Johns Hopkins University. Allegedly the KKI had been negligent in the way it conducted the study and specifically had breached its duty of care to the children by failing to notify their parents of their children's risk of lead exposure and other research risks. As pointed out by Joanne Pollak, legal counsel at Johns Hopkins, when the case reached Maryland's highest court "[t]here had been no trial on the facts in the lower court, including no exploration of the study design, the consent documents or the nature of the repair and maintenance measures in the homes" (p. 92).[20] Nonetheless, the court issued an opinion strongly critical of the institutional review board's (IRB) oversight of the research and set limits on the conduct of nontherapeutic research on children in Maryland. The opinion questions whether it is ethically permissible to conduct research on "less expensive, less effective" public health interventions when an effective but more expensive intervention is available, and if ethically permissible, what review and oversight and what decision-making processes should be required.[21]

Lead poisoning is a serious threat to the health and well-being of children. A major source of lead poisoning for children is living in a house with lead paint applied before 1978, when lead paint was banned in houses. The principal investigators in the KKI study, Mark Farfel and Julian Chisolm, had spent many years understanding and documenting the negative impacts of lead paint exposure on children's development. In the late 1980s, as described by Gerald Markowitz and David Rosner in their book *Lead Wars: The Politics of Science and the Fate of America's Children,* the political reality was "public health workers lacked political support for attaining the legislation and appropriations needed to end childhood [lead] poisoning. Yet the [lead] paint problem was enormous" (p. 145).[19] The KKI researchers were hoping to find acceptable ways to partially abate lead-based paint in housing so landlords would be willing to clean up rather than abandon their properties.

The KKI researchers designed their study to determine the effectiveness of three different levels of lead reduction in lessening children's exposure to lead paint and lead dust. They intended to compare the results of varying levels of lead reduction against two control groups living in previously abated houses. At the time, it cost about $20,000 to completely abate a house. The three partial abatement procedures cost $1,650, $3,500, $6,500, respectively.[21] The study apparently anticipated that some children might accumulate lead in their blood from exposure to dust because the researchers planned to take blood samples from the children at designated intervals, tracking the differences between the groups with different levels of exposure. Markowitz and Rosner point out that at the time the study was designed "determination of the relationship between lead in house dust and children's blood lead levels" was believed by lead researchers to be critical (p. 147).[19] Showing comparative effectiveness of their abatement strategy seemed to require a biological measure of measuring children's blood lead levels over a number of years.[19] The study was not considered an observational study because the researchers actively participated in the placement of families in the homes as well as abating conditions of the houses.

The Maryland Court of Appeals determined that the nature of "nontherapeutic" research (research that does not offer a treatment to the subjects) does potentially create a legal duty of care between a researcher and a research participant, a seminal finding that could permit a case of negligence to proceed against the researchers and their institutions. In legal terms, it gave rise to a special relationship in which such duties can arise. But because material questions of fact to support a negligence finding remained in dispute, the court sent the case back to a lower court for trial. The court also found the informed consent in the KKI study inadequate because the information that would be important to enable the parents to make a decision about whether or not to participate was not provided to the parents. Although KKI argued that all the children had a history of living in houses that contained lead, suggesting the researchers did not harm the children, the court's opinion concluded "[i]t can be argued that the researchers intended that the children be the canaries in the mines but never clearly told the parents" (p. 813).[18]

The court opinion also compared the abatement study with other significant research scandals. It stated, for example, that

> the research project at issue here, and its apparent protocols, differs in large degree from, but presents similar problems as those in the Tuskegee Syphilis Study, . . . the intentional exposure of soldiers to radiation in the 1940s and 1950s, . . . the tests involving the exposure of Navajo miners to radiation and the secret administration of LSD to soldiers by the CIA and the Army in the 1950s and 60s. (p. 816)[18]

The court continued by invoking other instances of abusive research including a reference to experiments conducted by the Nazis on inmates of concentration camps.[18]

Some have vigorously objected to the court's comparison of the partial lead abatement project to these other egregious studies because the KKI study did not intentionally deceive subjects or expose captive populations to harmful substances. Indeed, the study's ultimate aim was to learn how to reduce risks of exposure to lead paint. The study's defenders urge that the researchers' motivation was noble and benevolent and that low-income minority children in Baltimore were targeted because the children were most in need of improved housing. They argue that the research should have been undertaken because greater harm would result from denying to disadvantaged populations the benefits of potential improvement of living conditions that affect health.[21] Moreover, the children in the study were not exposed to any greater harm than they would have been if they had not been in the study. Finally, it is contended that the court's comparison is sensationalistic and ultimately harmful because it discourages other researchers from undertaking projects targeted to the needs of minorities and the poor. While the defenders of the study make important points, it should be noted such arguments do not address the question whether scientists or funding agencies are in the best position to decide exclusively, for example, that not going forward with proposed research would deny to disadvantaged populations the benefits of potential improvement in their lives.

Critics of the KKI study urge that the comparisons were on point and agree with the court's opinion, which observed that "[t]hese programs [of past egregious research] were somewhat alike in the vulnerability of the subjects. . . . . . .In the present case, children, especially young children, living in economic circumstances, albeit not as vulnerable as the other examples, are nonetheless, vulnerable as well" (p. 817).[18] As noted by Markowitz and Rosner, "[n]o one would suggest that a middle-class family allow their children to be knowingly exposed to a toxin that could be removed from their immediate environment" (p. 25).[19]

The court challenged the adequacy of the traditional regulatory and institutional system of ethics oversight in research, suggesting that IRBs are inherently biased toward the promotion of science and are not alone capable of making certain decisions: the opinion observes, "scientific and medical communities cannot be permitted to assume sole authority to determine ultimately what is right and appropriate in respect to research projects involving young children. . . . The Institutional Review Boards, IRBs, are primarily, in-house organs. . . . [T]hey are not designed . . . to be sufficiently objective in the sense that they are sufficiently concerned with the ethicality of the experiments they review as they are with the success of the experiments" (p. 817).[18] In this regard, the court suggested that the IRB encouraged the researchers to revise the IRB application so that the research would be characterized as therapeutic and therefore subject to a less rigorous standard of review.[18] Markowitz and Rosner note that the IRB head, Thomas Hendrix, assisted researchers with a key aspect of IRB review, offering suggestions about characterization of therapeutic benefit to children in control groups (living in lead-free housing) that presumably would minimize regulatory obstacles and increase the likelihood of IRB approval. He did not however offer specific guidance concerning potential harm to children living in partially abated homes.[19] Principal investigator Farfel responded to Hendrix indicating "that the study would have a separate consent form for each child and would include a section in the protocol that incorporated Hendrix's suggestions, redefining the potential benefits to the control groups" (p. 157).[19] Although the consent forms were revised, with respect to anticipated harm, the approved form merely said that "the repairs are not intended, or expected, to completely remove exposure to lead" (p. 158).[19] If the consent forms had been more detailed regarding crucial information about potential harm to children in homes with partial abatement, it is possible that the parents might not have agreed to participate in the study.

The options available to the parents and children in the KKI study were limited: they were not able to find affordable lead-free housing because of the paucity of such housing in Baltimore. They were also the very population that might benefit from the study's results. It is possible that some critics of the study might at some future time agree that appropriately designed less expensive, less effective but socially valuable public health intervention studies involving children could be ethically justified if there was broader consultation and involvement with those whom the research might likely benefit. It would be important, however, to address the knowledge and power disparities between researchers and subjects and their families. Researchers and research subjects may differ in their assessments of research benefits and risks. The subjects and their communities along with researchers and their institutions should seek consensus on the issue of whether research designed to reduce levels of lead dust in their homes or in their communities is potentially important enough to put themselves and their children at risk from participation in a research study.

A Contemporary Context for Research Involving African Americans

At the beginning of the twenty-first century, disparities between blacks and whites persist in every sector of American life, including health outcomes and health care. In 2002, the Institute of Medicine (IOM, now the National Academy of Medicine) issued a significant report, *Unequal Treatment: Confronting Racial and Ethnic Disparities in Health Care*, that recognized and documented black disadvantage in health care.[22] It found that racial and ethnic disparities in health care existed, often resulted in less effective care and occurred in the broader context of historic and persistent social and economic inequality.[22] Significantly, the report drew attention to additional sources of social inequities that suggested America is not yet a color-blind society. The report used circumstantial evidence to declare that bias, stereotyping, and prejudice were possible contributory factors of racial health disparities (Finding 4-1).[22] Today, increasing evidence supports that finding. Social psychologists Mahzarin Banaji and Anthony Greenwald in their book *Blindspot* describe these hidden biases as, "bits of knowledge [about social groups] . . . stored in our brains because we encounter them so frequently in our cultural environments. Once lodged in our minds, hidden biases can influence our behavior toward members of particular social groups, but we remain oblivious to their influence" (p. xii).[23] A number of studies have shown that such implicit race bias is pervasive[23] and support a conclusion that it impacts the health of blacks and their experiences with the health care system.[24]

In health research, classifying research subjects by race and ethnicity may provide valuable information about lifestyle, diet, or values that relate to health outcomes. Indeed, such information may uncover disparities in health outcomes and justify affirmative efforts to reduce or eliminate them. Yet focusing on perceived inherent racial differences still also risks promoting biological explanations for social inequalities in ways that make them seem natural. Continuing down this path risks naturalizing, reifying, and reinforcing social inequities.[25] To be clear, invoking biological explanations raises the danger of racism—the adverse, unjustified, and demeaning treatment of people on a simplistic view of race.

Moreover, false beliefs in biological differences may also lead to racial differences in health care. Two recent studies, one composed of lay white people and the other conducted with medical students and residents, find that a substantial number of participants hold false beliefs about biological differences between whites and blacks, (e.g., blacks have thicker skin or black people's blood coagulates more quickly than white people's blood). Significantly, this work also shows that those false beliefs predict racial bias in pain assessment and management.[26]

Finally, structural or regulatory arrangements in our major social institutions including health care and research institutions may also foster discrimination or disadvantage against blacks. Clearly, historically mandated segregation of blacks and whites in hospitals is an example of institutional discrimination. While civil rights laws have banned blatant forms of racism, institutional structures and procedures may still operate to further black disadvantage in health settings. For example, law professor Jonathan Kahn uses the story of BiDil® to illustrate how a confluence of institutional, legal, and commercial forces led to the federal Food and Drug Administration's (FDA)

2005 approval of the first drug with a race-specific indication for African Americans.[27] FDA undoubtedly believed that there was evidence to support the conclusion that BiDil worked better for African Americans with congestive heart failure. The agency might even have been influenced by the testimony of African Americans that in some small way its action could mitigate disparities between blacks and whites. There was certainly testimony from black patients and physicians that approving BiDil was important and beneficial to some members of the black community. Yet, BiDil's approval rested primarily on a study composed of African Americans only. In the absence of comparative data and mechanistic knowledge about how the drug works, it is inaccurate to represent BiDil as better or different in blacks than in whites. BiDil may work for some people with congestive heart failure, but who might benefit cannot be determined by reference to self-identified race.[28] Unfortunately, FDA approval of BiDil with a race-specific indication suggests that race is based in biological differences.[29]

Looking Ahead

To successfully combat the force of historical and contemporary stereotypes, bias, and disadvantage, policymakers and researchers need a conception of justice to guide choices and behaviors about how to interact with patients, about what research questions to ask, about whom to include in studies, and about how to include them.

The first national effort to come up with a framework for ethics in biomedical research, the National Commission for the Protection of Human Subjects of Biomedical and Behavioral Research (of which the author was a member) (National Commission), was convened in 1974 to respond in part to revelations about the treatment of black research subjects in the Tuskegee Syphilis Study. The National Commission's recommendations became the basis for subsequently promulgated federal regulations setting out requirements for ethical participation of human subjects in biomedical research.

The National Commission's *Belmont Report*[30] set forth its conception of justice as "fairness in distribution." By that it meant that in order to treat individual persons and social groups as equals, the research community needed to distribute both the burdens and benefits of research in a fair manner. Such a fair distribution demanded in particular "fair procedures and outcomes in the selection of subjects" at both the social and the individual level:

> Individual justice in the selection of subjects would require that researchers exhibit fairness: thus, they should not offer potentially beneficial research only to some patients who are in their favor or select

only "undesirable" persons for risky research. Social justice requires that a distinction be drawn between classes of subjects that ought, and ought not, to participate in any particular kind of research, based on the ability of members of that class to bear burdens and on the appropriateness of placing further burdens on already burdened persons . . . Injustice may appear in the selection of subjects, even if individual subjects are selected fairly by investigators and treated fairly in the course of research. (p. 23196)[30]

The National Commission issued several reports on specific groups (e.g., children, fetuses, prisoners) with requirements for obtaining informed consent and specified procedures for assessing the risk to which research subjects could be exposed. Those reports reflected the National Commission's sense of the fair allocation of research burdens and benefits for those groups. Notably, the National Commission did not provide specific guidance for fair inclusion of racial and ethnic minorities or economically and educationally disadvantaged persons.

In 1984, the US Department of Health and Human Services established the Task Force on Black and Minority Health to ascertain available knowledge of the health status of blacks and other minorities.[31] The Task Force's Report issued in 1985 marked a shift in the federal government's attitude toward black health status. The report documented racial disparities in health status, noted the absence of data about many aspects of minority health and called for greater inclusion of racial and ethnic minorities in medical research.[32] In 1993, the United States Congress enacted the NIH Revitalization Act of 1993 (P.L. 103-43) to promote inclusion of minorities (and women) in federally funded clinical research. The legislation required self-identified racial and ethnic characteristics of research participants be collected, categorized, and recorded in research documentation in accordance with the federal Office of Management and Budget definition of racial and ethnic groups.[33]

In the contemporary research context that emphasizes inclusion of vulnerable groups, the distributive paradigm put forth by the National Commission needs to be reexamined. The *Belmont Report*'s articulation of the principle of justice though concerned with protection does not provide adequate guidance for inclusion of historically disadvantaged groups. That report does mention racial minorities in discussions of the principle of justice, specifically in its discussion of selection of research subjects and unfair distributions of the burdens and benefits of research. The report states,

. . . the selection of research subjects needs to be scrutinized in order to determine whether some classes (e.g., welfare patients, particular racial and ethnic minorities, or persons confined to institutions) are being systematically selected simply because of their easy availability, their compromised position, or their manipulability, rather than for reasons directly related to the problem being studied. (p. 23194)[30]

Current regulations governing research with human subjects that find their ethical justification in the *Belmont Report* do not establish guidelines for research with economically and educationally disadvantaged research subjects.[34] Today, African Americans deserve a moral framework that attends to their lack of power in their dealings with researchers and physicians, that appreciates the need to move away from reliance on biological explanations for difference, and that challenges newer forms of disadvantage such as the prevalence of racial bias in a purportedly race-blind society.

Iris Marion Young, for example, offers a compelling view of an appropriate conception of justice that incorporates and moves beyond the distribution paradigm. Young argues that concepts of domination and oppression should be the starting point for a conception of justice. She contends with two flaws in the distribution paradigm. "First, it tends to focus thinking about social justice on the allocation of material goods such as things, resources, income, and wealth or on the distribution of social positions, especially jobs. This focus tends to ignore the social structure and institutional context that often help to determine distributive patterns" (p. 15).[35] Young wants to highlight issues of decision-making, division of labor, and culture that are important to a conception of justice but are ignored in distributive justice discussions. Although Young acknowledges that it is possible to use the distributive paradigm in distribution of nonmaterial goods, she makes a second point: "When metaphorically extended to nonmaterial goods [(e.g., rights, opportunity, power and self-respect)], the concept of distribution represents them as though they were static things, instead of a function of social relations and processes" (p. 16).[35] In Young's words, "[w]ithout a structural understanding of power and domination as processes rather than patterns of distribution, the existence and nature of domination and oppression in these societies cannot be identified" (p. 33).[35]

Domination is concerned with institutional conditions, which inhibit or prevent persons from being self-determining, developing one's capacities, or expressing one's experiences. "Persons live within structures of domination if . . . [others] can determine . . . the conditions of their action, either directly or by virtue of the structural consequences of their actions" (p. 38).[35] According to Young, "oppression . . . refers to systemic constraints on groups . . . Oppression in this sense is structural . . . Its causes are embedded in unquestioned norms, habits, and symbols, in the assumptions underlying institutional rules and the collective consequences in following those rules" (p. 41).[35] Groups that are dominant establish their own rules as the norm and mark other groups and their perspectives as invisible and deviant and mark those who hold them as "the Other." Young emphasizes the importance of social context and the significance of power in relationships thus underscoring the need for change in the institutions and conditions under which inequality arises. Finally, it should be stressed that changing the conditions of inequality also requires addressing interlocking systems of subordination—sex, race, and class—that are complex and diverse in their interactions with those who have power in the society.

It is critically important that African Americans participate in research, even in the shadow of past abuses in medicine and research and the distrust those abuses have fostered, and even though, as currently designed, biomedical research relies on race while trying to broaden the inclusion of African Americans in research. African American participation is necessary for at least two reasons. First, diversifying all institutions of our society including all aspects of our health and medical enterprise is an important path for achieving justice for all marginalized persons. African Americans should not forget the past but they also should not allow the memories to become an obstacle to achieving benefits in the present.

Second, biomedical research offers the prospect of reducing racial disparities in health and health care and for developing treatments for disease and adverse conditions. Participation is especially important at this time because of President Obama's 2015 Precision Medicine Initiative (subsequently referred to as the "All of Us Research Program").[36,37] The goal of the initiative is for researchers, providers, and patients to work together to develop individualized care.[37] Without such participation African Americans miss an opportunity to advance research on factors especially relevant to African American health. Although increased African American participation in research could have a profound effect on African American health status in the future, it will not come about unless barriers to participation are also addressed.

Just as today's trends in clinical research and medicine should be informed by historical knowledge, so a conception of justice must be sensitive to and steeped in marginalized communities' experiences with and attitudes toward medicine and biomedical research. The historical and contemporary case studies described above—the Tuskegee Syphilis Study, the experiences of Henrietta Lacks and her family, the Baltimore lead abatement study, the discussions around approval of BiDil, and others—deserve reflection in reconsideration of the distributive paradigm in research and efforts to increase African American participation in research.

The KKI study was subject to review and oversight under federal regulations that were promulgated in response to the National Commission's *Belmont Report* and other recommendations. Indeed the *Grimes* court thought that Johns Hopkins University's IRB had abdicated its responsibilities by advising investigators to amend the protocol so that the researchers would not have to meet the stringent requirements attached to nontherapeutic research with children.[18] The court's statements about the IRB suggest concerns about professional self-regulation and research bureaucracy that should be taken seriously. In reality, IRBs must attempt to strike a delicate balance between advancing science and protecting research subjects. Achieving this balance is especially a concern when evaluating the risks, benefits, and study design of research on vulnerable populations, especially when the intended subjects are made vulnerable in multiple ways by race and ethnicity, by age, and by class. As mentioned previously, IRBs may need additional guidance for research involving the poor and the vulnerable. In addition, IRB members as well as researchers may need targeted education and training to increase awareness of unconscious bias and its possible impact on decision-making. The very fact that our implicit bias is hidden from our consciousness is an indication that raising such awareness needs explicit attention.

The families in the KKI study were part of a broader community of similarly situated families who were underserved and vulnerable. The researchers' good intentions not withstanding in these circumstances, it might have behooved the researchers, even if not the standard practice at the time, to engage proactively with the broader community in designing a partial lead abatement study that met the needs and values of all stakeholders. Social psychologist Phillip Bowman urges that in addition to ethical and scientific guidelines "research among racial minorities . . . must be guided by principles of *significant involvement and functional relevance*. In this context, *significant involvement* calls for the members of the group under study to have a central role in the entire research process. Functional relevance dictates that studies should operate to promote the needs and perspectives of the study population" (p. 754).[38] Involvement of stakeholders and communities is a means of acknowledging that focus on the individual patient or subject does not take sufficient account of the individual's history and context, thus obscuring important considerations of social justice and distrust.

Today greater attention is directed to involving the ways in which communities can participate as partners in research, particularly in the recruitment of subjects. Collaboration in efforts to establish the research agenda and the research protocol itself is also warranted. A research oversight model that focuses on informed consent and IRB oversight may not be sufficient to protect those who have suffered from past injustice and are educationally and economically disadvantaged. For example, some proposals for increased enrollment of African Americans in research have called for community involvement in recruitment. Community involvement is desirable because it helps to empower participants. We can only speculate that with early and broad input from the communities in which the children lived, the KKI study might not have been challenged. Mari Matsuda reminds us that those with little power see the world they live in differently from those who have power, so that the experiences, history, and culture of people of color constitute a valuable epistemological source.[39] The involvement of the Lacks family members in reviewing research involving the HeLa cells is an important development and hopefully will serve as a model for future interactions between researchers and research participants.

Although many believe that the disclosure of the Tuskegee Syphilis Study in 1972 is the source of African Americans' ongoing distrust of medical professionals and their health care and research institutions, the seeds of distrust go back to slavery. As Brandt explains, "[t]he Tuskegee Study reveals the persistence of beliefs within the medical profession about the nature of blacks, sex, and disease—beliefs that had tragic repercussions long after their alleged 'scientific' bases were known to be incorrect" (p. 27).[5] The study also confirmed for African Americans historical patterns of abuse that have been orally passed down through generations. Even today the term "night doctors," discussed previously in connection with the Lacks family, continues to be used. Medical professionals need to understand why they are distrusted and why this distrust persists today. Medical professionals must also appreciate that stereotypes and bias persist in the profession and may be manifested in medical interactions with African Americans.

The African American community also has responsibility to address this mistrust. Myths and rumors, though often connected to past events, need to be addressed by community leaders. The National Bioethics Center at Tuskegee University and the pharmaceutical company Eli Lilly, for example, have announced a collaboration to develop a plan that would work toward increasing African American participation in clinical trials.[40]

Despite many examinations of the legacy of the Tuskegee Syphilis Study, it is not clear whether the dangers of its reliance on biological explanations to explain differences between blacks and whites is fully appreciated today. As historian Susan Reverby explains, "BiDil and Tuskegee demonstrate the problems of ignoring individuals by using race as a proxy and of remembering Tuskegee only in terms of racism. It is the 'logic' of race, not just acts of racism that undergirded Tuskegee . . . which demands recognition" (pp. 478–479).[29]

In fact, the widespread use of race in medical and scientific research has spawned a vigorous debate about its appropriateness. African Americans' interests in better health and health care should not be put at risk while this debate continues without resolution. A recent article recommends that "[t]he U.S. National Academies of Sciences, Engineering, and Medicine should convene a panel of experts from the biological sciences, social sciences, and humanities to recommend ways for research into human biological diversity to move past the use of race as a tool for classification in both laboratory and clinical research" (p. 565).[41] The authors recommend further that the committee's charge be to examine "current and historical usage of the race concept and ways current and future technology might improve the study of human genetic diversity" (p. 565).[41] This is an important recommendation. Racial terminology should be phased out and the best way to accomplish that goal is to appeal to our most significant and credible scientific institutions.

Conclusion

The work of involving African Americans and other minorities in the research enterprise is important and ongoing. This chapter has briefly examined three controversial examples of African American participation in the twentieth-century research because it is important to focus on the human settings in which injustice and ethical dilemmas are embedded and experienced. Appreciation of past injustice is relevant to the present as these examples of African American participation in research illustrate. A shared discussion and retelling of historical injustice provides an avenue for people of different perspectives, racial and ethnic backgrounds, and social class an opportunity to develop mutual respect. More importantly, understanding how past injustices connect to the present uncovers how structural impediments to achieving just conditions in the present evolved and may offer clues about what modifications in the present might be effective. Finally, understanding and acknowledging the interrelationships between past injustice and the present gives additional weight to moral arguments for making changes in the present not only for African Americans but also for other minorities and marginalized groups as well.

Acknowledgment

I would like to thank Anna Mastroianni for her invaluable organization, editorial and technical assistance contributions, and without whom it would have been impossible to complete this chapter.

Notes

1. Plous S, Williams T. Racial stereotypes from the days of American slavery: a continuing legacy. *Journal of Applied Social Psychology*. 1995;25(9):795–817.
2. Jones J. *Bad Blood: The Tuskegee Syphilis Experiment*. New York, NY: Free Press; 1981.
3. Lerner BH, Caplan AL. Judging the past: how history should inform bioethics. *Annals of Internal Medicine*. 2016;164(8):553–557.
4. DuBois WEB. The health and physique of the Negro American, 1906. *American Journal of Public Health*. 2003;93(2):272–276.
5. Brandt AM. Racism and research: the case of the Tuskegee Syphilis Study. *Hastings Center Report*. 1978;8(6):21–29.
6. Higginbotham EB. African-American women's history and the metalanguage of race. *Signs*. 1992;17(2):251–274.
7. Tuskegee Syphilis Study Ad hoc Advisory Panel. *Final Report*. Washington, DC: US Department of Health, Education and Welfare; 1973.
8. Skloot R. *The Immortal Life of Henrietta Lacks*. New York, NY: Crown Publishers; 2010.
9. Fett SM. *Working Cures: Healing, Health, and Power on Southern Slave Plantations*. Chapel Hill, NC: University of North Carolina Press; 2002.
10. Fry G-M. *Night Riders in Black Folk History*. Chapel Hill, NC: University of North Carolina Press; 2001.
11. Public Broadcasting Service. Baltimore hospitals work to repair frayed trust in black communities. *PBS Newshour*. PBS television. February 15, 2016. http://www.pbs.org/newshour/bb/baltimore-hospitals-work-to-repair-frayed-trust-in-black-communities/. Accessed December 4, 2017.
12. Hancock J; Kaiser Health News. In Freddie Gray's neighborhood, the best medical care is close but elusive. http://khn.org/news/in-freddie-grays-neighborhood-the-best-medical-care-is-close-but-elusive/. Published February 16, 2016. Accessed December 4, 2017.
13. Landecker H. *Culturing Life: How Cells Became Technologies*. Cambridge, MA: Harvard University Press; 2007.
14. Fee E. Sin vs. science: venereal disease in Baltimore in the Twentieth Century. *The Journal of the History of Medicine and Allied Sciences*. 1988;43(2):141–164.
15. Landecker H. Immortality, in vitro: a history of the HeLa cell line. In: Brodwin PE, ed. *Biotechnology and Culture: Bodies, Anxieties, Ethics*. Bloomington, IN: Indiana University Press; 2000:53–72.

16. NIH, Lacks family reach understanding to share genomic data of HeLa cells [news release]. Bethesda, MD: National Institutes of Health; August 7, 2013. http://www.nih.gov/news-events/news-releases/nih-lacks-family-reach-understanding-share-genomic-data-hela-cells. Accessed December 4, 2017.

17. Hudson KL, Collins FS. Biospecimen policy: family matters. *Nature*. 2013;500(7461):141–142.

18. *Grimes v. Kennedy Krieger Institute, Inc.*, 782 A.2d 807 (2001).

19. Markowitz G, Rosner D. *Lead Wars: The Politics of Science and the Fate of America's Children*. Berkeley, CA: University of California Press; 2013.

20. Pollak J. The lead-based abatement repair and maintenance study in Baltimore: historic framework and study design. *Journal of Health Care Law & Policy*. 2002;6(1):89–108.

21. Buchanan DR, Miller FG. Justice and Fairness in the Kennedy Krieger Institute lead paint study: the ethics of public health research on less expensive, less effective interventions. *American Journal of Public Health*. 2006;96(5):781–787.

22. Smedley BD, Stith AY, Nelson AR, eds. *Unequal Treatment: Confronting Racial and Ethnic Disparities in Health Care*. Washington DC: National Academies Press; 2003.

23. Banaji MR, Greenwald AG. *Blindspot: The Hidden Biases of Good People*. New York, NY: Delacorte Press; 2013.

24. Green AR, Carney DR, Pallin DJ, et al. Implicit bias among physicians and its prediction of thrombolysis decisions for black and white patients. *Journal of General Internal Medicine*. 2007;22(9):1231–238.

25. Hammonds EM; Social Science Research Council. Straw men and their followers: the return of biological race [Web Forum]. http://raceandgenomics.ssrc.org/Hammonds/. Published June 7, 2006. Accessed December 4, 2017.

26. Hoffman KM, Trawalter S, Axt JR, Oliver MN. Racial bias in pain assessment and treatment recommendations, and false beliefs about biological differences between blacks and whites. *Proceedings of the National Academy of Sciences of the United States of America*. 2016;113(16):4296–4301.

27. Kahn J. *Race in a Bottle: The Story of Bidil and Racialized Medicine in a Post-Genomic Age*. New York, NY: Columbia University Press; 2013.

28. Krimsky S. The art of medicine: the short life of a race drug. *The Lancet*. 2012;379(9811):114–115.

29. Reverby SM. "Special treatment": BiDil, Tuskegee and the logic of race. *Journal of Law, Medicine & Ethics*. 2008;36 (3):478–484.

30. National Commission for the Protection of Human Subjects of Biomedical and Behavioral Research. The Belmont Report: Ethical principles and guidelines for the protection of human subjects of research. *Federal Register*. 1979;44(76):23192–23197.

31. Heckler MM. *Report of the Secretary's Task Force on Black and Minority Health*. Vols. 1–7. Washington, DC: US Department of Health and Human Services; 1985.

32. Savitt TL. Minorities as research subjects. In: Reich WT, ed. *Encyclopedia of Bioethics*. 2nd ed. Vol. 3. New York, NY: Simon & Schuster Macmillan; 1995:1776–1780.

33. National Institutes of Health. NIH policy and guidelines on the inclusion of women and minorities as subjects in clinical research—amended, October, 2001. https://grants.nih.gov/grants/funding/women_min/guidelines_amended_10_2001.htm. Accessed December 4, 2017.

34. Stone TH. The invisible vulnerable: the economically and educationally disadvantaged subjects of clinical research. *Journal of Law, Medicine & Ethics*. 2003;31(1):149–153.

35. Young IM. *Justice and the Politics of Difference*. Princeton, NJ: Princeton University Press; 1990.

36. The White House. Fact sheet: President Obama's Precision Medicine Initiative [press release]. Washington, DC: The White House; January, 30, 2015. https://www.whitehouse.gov/the-press-office/2015/01/30/fact-sheet-president-obama-s-precision-medicine-initiative. Accessed December 4, 2017.

37. National Institutes of Health All of Us Research Program Website. https://allofus.nih.gov/. Accessed December 4, 2017.

38. Bowman PJ. Race, class and ethics in research: *Belmont* principles to functional relevance. In: Jones RJ, ed. *Black Psychology*. 3rd ed. Berkeley, CA: Cobb & Henry Publishers; 1991:747–766.

39. Matsuda MJ. Looking to the bottom: critical legal studies and reparations. *Harvard Civil Rights-Civil Liberties Law Review*. 1987;22(1):323–399.

40. Tuskegee University. Tuskegee University and Eli Lilly and Company collaborate to enhance African American participation in clinical trials [press release]. http://tuskegeebioethics.org/african-americans-lilly-clinical-trials-news-release/. Published February 23, 2016. Accessed December 4, 2017.

41. Yudell M, Roberts D, DeSalle R, Tishkoff S. Taking race out of human genetics. *Science*. 2016;351(6237):564–565.

8 JUSTICE, RESEARCH, AND COMMUNITIES

Katherine F. King
James V. Lavery

Biomedical research ethics have historically focused on the rights, interests, and welfare of individual research subjects. For instance, according to Robert Levine, the National Commission for the Protection of Human Subjects in Biomedical and Behavioral Research seemed "to embrace an atomistic view of the person. . . . Except, perhaps, in its report on research involving children, there is little or no reference to persons in relationship to others or as members of communities" (p. 13).[1] However, over the past twenty years, investigators, funders, and sponsors have increasingly recognized that communities can be harmed and benefited by research.

The growing emphasis on engaging communities in research, and on-going efforts to increase the participation of communities in research, have, to a significant extent, grown out of moral concerns about justice in biomedical research. Notable issues include who gets to decide what research is conducted with or on communities, what constitutes a fair distribution of risks, burdens, and benefits in research, and who has the authority to speak for a community about these issues. Consider, for example, genetic research and HIV prevention research.

Research into the genetic basis of breast and ovarian cancer revealed that mutations in the BRCA1 and BRCA2 genes, which increase the risk of women developing breast or ovarian cancer, are more prevalent among Ashkenazi Jews in the United States than in the wider US population. This raised concerns that the research findings would be used to discriminate against all Ashkenazi Jews, particularly around access to health insurance.[2] The early research into these genes used an existing collection of de-identified tissue samples.[3] As a result, an institutional review board (IRB) determined that the study represented minimal risk to those individuals who originally contributed the samples, and therefore did not require their informed consent. Many in the Jewish community rejected this decision, pointing out that the research could harm them by increasing the potential for stigma and decreasing access to insurance.[3] The 2008 US Genetic Information Non-Discrimination Act was subsequently passed to protect individuals against health insurance and employment discrimination on the basis of genetic information. However, discrimination in the purchase of other forms of insurance, particularly long-term care insurance, life insurance, or disability insurance, remains a worry for members of many communities that are known to be at higher risk of having a particular disease or condition.[4]

Another example concerns a case of HIV prevention research. In 2003, a team of researchers from the University of California at San Francisco approached sex workers in Phnom Pen, Cambodia, about participating in a trial assessing whether the use of tenofovir disoproxil fumarate (tenofovir) as preexposure prophylaxis (PrEP) could prevent HIV transmission. While the researchers made efforts to engage the community of sex workers, the trial was closed prematurely in the face of substantial public backlash in support of the sex workers.[5-7] The factors contributing to the closure are complex, but one major consideration was the failure to establish meaningful communication between the research team and the sex workers. Although the research team held many community meetings and established a community advisory board (CAB), the sex-worker community reported that they did not feel listened to or understood by the researchers, nor did they feel that their concerns about safety and the lack of guarantees about compensation for research-related harms were taken seriously.[6,8] As a result, the sex-worker community voiced their issues in the international press and the trial was ultimately shut down.

In this chapter, we take a closer look at how the history and practice of community engagement in research has highlighted questions of justice and the wider social implications of biomedical research beyond a focus on individual research subjects. *Community engagement* (CE) includes the broad set of practices that help researchers establish and maintain relationships with the research community for a specific study to advance a range of ethical and practical goals. CE includes, but is not limited to, CABs, direct engagement with a wide range of stakeholders, and various forms of participatory research. These CE strategies differ in how they structure the relationship between the community and the researcher, but share a core moral motivation of giving a voice to the community in the conduct of research.

Justice Over Time

In this section, we provide a historical view on communities in biomedical research, focusing, in particular, on the role of HIV/AIDS advocacy in bringing the importance of communities to biomedical research to public attention. We then consider the moral foundation for engaging with communities in research, discuss issues related to defining communities, and then look at three primary models that have emerged to structure relationships between researchers and communities.

The Call for Community Engagement

In the United States, attention to the role of communities in research emerged during the early history of HIV/AIDS research in the 1980s. During those early days, HIV/AIDS advocates reframed access to research as a matter of justice for the HIV/AIDS community as a whole. They argued that participation in research offered significant benefits, and in many cases was the only source of potentially beneficial treatment, despite the emphasis on risk to individual research participants associated with the new HIV treatments being tested. As a result, access to and oversight of research activities were a matter of justice, and that they, as a community, should have a greater voice in the conduct of research, from defining research priorities to shaping trial design and overseeing its implementation.

This activism led to the formation of the first CAB in 1988, which formalized the involvement of the community in the research process.[9] The following year, the National Institute of Allergy and Infectious Disease (NIAID) of the US National Institutes of Health (NIH) required CABs as a condition of funding of HIV/AIDS trials, providing an opportunity for community input on the design and implementation of clinical trials. The NIH continues to require community representation in all of the HIV/AIDS research that it funds, and has built up a network of CABs and community representatives operating at individual trial sites, at the level of clinical trial networks, and across such networks.[10] These programs have given rise to a unique culture of community participation in HIV research.

The HIV/AIDS community has also led international advocacy efforts around community involvement in research. In particular, UNAIDS (Joint United Nations Programme on HIV/AIDS), in collaboration with the AIDS Vaccine Advocacy Coalition (AVAC), has played a vitally important role in establishing CE as an accepted component of all population-based HIV clinical trials globally through the development and implementation of the Good Participatory Practice Guidelines (GPP).[11] The guidelines were first issued in 2007 and updated in 2011, and have become the primary guidance for engaging communities in HIV–related research. The guidelines highlight the importance of both informal stakeholder engagement activities (such as local events, focus group discussions, interviews, or consultations) to more formal activities aimed at developing an ongoing relationship with the community at a particular trial site (such as CABs). They have also defined expectations for CE beyond research in HIV/AIDS. Recently, the guidelines were adapted to research in tuberculosis,[12] and the US President's Commission for the Study of Bioethical Issues (PCSBI) highlighted them as a model for CE across all biomedical research.[13]

While HIV/AIDS research brought CE into the spotlight in biomedical research, it has also become standard practice in other areas of biomedical research.

Research with Aboriginal Populations

Research with aboriginal populations in North America was one of the first domains of biomedical research to require CE. Since the 1970s in the United States, the Indian Health Services has required prior approval by the local tribal government for all human subjects research.[14] Similarly, the Canadian Tri-Council Policy Statement requires engagement in biomedical research with First Nations, Inuit, and Métis populations and offers comprehensive guidance on how researchers and communities should go about the engagement process.[15] Requirements to engage with aboriginal populations reflect the history of these communities in North America, and in particular, it speaks to the need to counter the historical context of exploitation, marginalization, and distrust.

Genetic Research

In 1999, the US National Bioethics Advisory Commission (NBAC) recommended community consultation for population-level genetic research in which the outcomes of the research could harm members of the population from which the samples were collected by contributing to stigmatization or discrimination against the group.[16] While NBAC did not recommend specific mechanisms of engagement, it argued that the researchers should seek to understand the nature of the risks presented by the research to the community as well as strategies to mitigate those risks.[16] CE has subsequently become integrated into most population-level genetic research and genetic database research initiatives.[17-20]

Institutional Approaches

Most recently, the NIH has required CE for all institutions receiving funding under the Clinical and Translational Science Awards (CTSA) Program.[21] These awards require recipients to establish core CE services to foster long-term, bidirectional relationships between the institution and communities.[22] The CTSA approach differs from the previous examples of CE by requiring engagement at the level of the recipient institution, rather than with individual research projects or research networks. Early research suggests that institutions are adopting a wide range of strategies to build relationships with the community.[22] This includes educational initiatives about CE for investigators, institutional staff, and community members; the development of CABs and involvement of community members on expert panels; and public announcements and notifications about research activities at the institution.

Research in General

There is increasing awareness that CE practices are relevant and valuable in a wide range of biomedical research settings. For example, the US Centers for Disease Control and Prevention has highlighted the importance of CE for a wide range of public health programs and capacity building initiatives, as well as biomedical research programs.[21] Furthermore, formalized CE is now required for research in the emergency setting (see Chapter 3). Thus, there is a growing appreciation of the moral significance of CE practices throughout a wide range of research activities.

Moral Foundations

Historical attention to engaging communities in research arose from community activists who raised fundamental concerns about justice in research. Their voices called into question the familiar, somewhat narrow, ethical obligations of research and led to a reconsideration of these obligations, placing them within a social context that highlights issues of justice.

Identifying Nonobvious Risks and Benefits

CE is an important mechanism to help identify nonobvious risks and benefits of research for both individual research participants and the wider research community.[10–11,13,21,23–24] In evaluating research, investigators, IRBs, sponsors, and funders already consider a wide range of potential risks and benefits. However, what constitutes a risk, which risks are deemed to be acceptable, and by whom, are all influenced by the social, cultural, political, and economic circumstances that prevail in any given research context. Some of these risks may not be evident to researchers, particularly when conducting research with communities whose language, culture, and history are different from the researchers', nor are they likely to be immediately evident to the potential research participants themselves.

Rather, appreciation of the risks created by research accumulates through ongoing communications in the context of relationships with a range of stakeholders. Over time, communities come to appreciate the implications of research for them, and researchers can develop a deeper understanding of the potentially nonobvious ways in which their actions may affect the interests of the research community, as well as pathways through which these interests may be protected and satisfied.[11,25–26] CE supports this understanding by creating the infrastructure for sustained interaction with communities.

For example, in the tenofovir PrEP trials in Cambodia mentioned earlier, the local sex-worker community charged that the research staff failed to listen to their concerns about the risks and burdens of the trial and the inadequacy of the benefits. In particular, they argued that the trial staff did not recognize that their families relied on their income for survival. Missing work due to the adverse effects of the trial medication was a significant hardship, which, they argued, was inadequately offset by the benefits of research participation.

In a different case, the Havasupai tribe of Arizona brought a lawsuit against Arizona State University and some of its affiliated researchers in 2004. The tribe charged that the university researchers had inappropriately used blood samples of tribal members. The samples had originally been obtained for research on diabetes, a condition that is prevalent in the tribe. The researchers, however, also used the samples for three other studies involving the genetic basis of schizophrenia, inbreeding within the population, and the evolutionary genetics of the population.[27] Each of these three studies was seen as harmful to the community *by the community*—either by stigmatizing it or by undermining deeply held beliefs and cultural traditions, such as challenging origin beliefs. Ultimately, Arizona State University acknowledged this harm in a settlement that included a formal apology, return of blood samples to the community, and financial compensation.[27]

Extending "Respect" Beyond the Individual

Respect for research participants is central to research ethics. In the case of individuals, respect is understood largely as respect for the autonomy of research participants, and researchers meet this obligation largely through informed consent processes through which potential participants are given the opportunity to exercise their autonomous choice about participating in research. When applied to communities, the concept of respect is concerned with acknowledging communities and their authority to participate in decisions that affect them. In particular, it is possible to distinguish two important aspects of the concept of respect. First, respecting communities involves recognizing or acknowledging them as having legitimate interests in the research. Second, it involves providing them with the opportunity to influence, and ultimately to accept or reject, research participation.

To understand how CE contributes to respecting research communities, it is necessary to step back from the emphasis on informed consent as a mechanism for respecting individuals in biomedical research and return to the core of the concept.[28–31] In particular, respect is fundamentally a matter of acknowledging others. When extended to the context of research, respect includes acknowledging what is valuable, important, or risky about research to the research participants, and then acting in ways that express that recognition.[26,31] This understanding of *respect as acknowledgment or recognition* is central to CE. For example, the GPP guidelines argue that "respect is demonstrated when stakeholders communicate and act in ways that value and honor each other's perspectives and realities." (Section 2.1).[11] Similarly, the PCSBI argued CE respects communities by being responsive to local cultures,[13] and Emanuel and colleagues argue that respect in research with developing countries includes "recognition of and respect for the host community's distinctive values, culture, and social practices" by reflecting these issues in the design and implementation of the research study (p. 932).[32]

To some extent, the obligation to recognize the interests of research communities is already captured by the obligation to minimize risks to research participants. What is added by recognizing this broader obligation of respect is the recognition that the potential harm to research participants is broader than discrete risks. It also includes harms to their sense of their value and social standing that can result when researchers disregard or fail to listen to their interests and perspectives.

Indeed, the failure to listen to and acknowledge the concerns of stakeholders has been one of the most pronounced critiques levied against researchers by communities, particularly in the context of global health. This was a primary critique of the participants in the failed tenofovir PrEP trials in Cambodia discussed earlier.[6–7] In particular, when sex-workers raised questions about the conduct of the trial, they reported that the questions were interpreted as if they had a lack of understanding. As a result the trial staff responded by re-explaining the issue rather than initiating a discussion to explore the sex-worker's questions. This case underlines how difficult it can be to acknowledge community concerns. The researchers did engage communities procedurally: they held community meetings and formed a CAB. Nevertheless, the community was unsatisfied. Evaluating the effectiveness of engagement and the quality of communication between researchers and communities remains a significant challenge, which we will return to at the end of this chapter.[6–7]

Legitimacy

Acknowledgment of communities is insufficient if their voices and perspectives do not have real bearing on the conduct of research. CE seeks not only to give voice to the perspectives and concerns of the research community, but also to institute a process through which the conduct of research can become legitimate in the eyes of that community.[26] Broadly speaking, legitimacy is a dimension of justice that speaks to how authority over groups of people is justified. By imposing risks, as well as potential benefits, on groups and individuals, biomedical research raises questions of legitimacy. CE responds to these considerations by creating the opportunities for communities to accept or reject participation in the research project, while also increasing transparency, accountability, and, ultimately, trust between the community and the research team. As the PCSBI emphasized, these activities do not always have to change the direction of research to be meaningful:

> True community engagement provides opportunities for ongoing oversight and monitoring of the research activities. While this might not alter the scientific approach, it is an important political consideration because it allows communities to protect themselves and become invested in the ethical and valid conduct of the research. (p. 27)[33]

Defining Communities

The ability of CE to address these ethical concerns depends, to a large extent, on the structure of the relationships between the community and the researchers, including both how the research community is understood by researchers and by the members of that community, and how relationships with that community are organized.

Understanding who belongs to a research community is one of the most challenging aspects of respecting communities. The conventional view about research communities is that they correspond to preexisting associations of people. Very often, these communities are understood in terms of local neighborhoods, villages, or towns, but they also can be defined through a wide range of characteristics that bring people together, including ethnic, cultural, and religious identity, and common professions, among others.[34] As a result of these shared characteristics, communities, and not just individuals, could be exposed to risk through research, and the argument is that research protections should be extended to them.

The difficulty in practice is that this understanding of "community" refers to a wide array of human associations and groupings with varying degrees of organization, and as a result, there is no straightforward approach to linking the relevant research protections with the organization of these communities.[34] Some of the communities relevant to biomedical research, such as "disease communities," are very loosely organized with no legitimate political authority and have varying degrees of communication and shared culture and perspectives. However, other recognized communities, such as aboriginal communities, are highly organized and do have legitimate political authorities, a strong, shared culture, an organized economy, and established communication networks. In other cases, the community affected by a research program does not correspond to any preexisting community, but rather it is research activities themselves that coalesce the community.

To accommodate this diversity, a new understanding of the communities relevant to biomedical research has emerged.[10–12,21] On this approach, the research community consists of those groups and individuals who are stakeholders in the research, meaning that they have a legitimate interest in the conduct and outcomes of the research.[26] It is the presence of these shared interests in the conduct and outcomes of the research, with consequent shared risks, that defines the stakeholder community and grounds the moral responsibility for engagement with it.

The stakeholder approach to the research community leads to a very expansive view of research communities that includes not only traditional research participants, but also organizations and institutions within a local village as well as broader stakeholders such as local, national, and global nongovernmental organizations, policymakers, regulators, medical professionals, foundations, and funders.

Forms of Engagement

The relationship between researchers and communities also significantly influences the quality of engagement and the extent to which it addresses the moral concerns raised. There are three major approaches to organizing relationships with research communities: participatory research, CABs, and direct engagement.

Participatory Research

Participatory research refers to a diverse set of methods that emphasize the importance of bringing the community, including the beneficiaries, users, and stakeholders of the research, into the design, implementation, and dissemination of research.[35] These strategies are distinct from other forms of engagement in viewing the community as central to the knowledge production process. In particular, the goal of these methods is to integrate the practical, lived experience of the stakeholders with the theoretical and methodological knowledge of researcher partners to produce knowledge that is more readily translated into improved practice.

Participatory research strategies tend to have an explicit emphasis on social empowerment. Community participation aims to enable empowerment of individuals, organizations, and communities by building a shared understanding of problems, and collaborative, coordinated action to address those problems.[36] The community groups involved may be marginalized, and the research process itself is structured to support empowerment by minimizing power differentials between the community and researchers and democratizing the knowledge production process by recognizing community members as equal partners. However, the extent to which these outcomes are actually achieved through participatory research practices remains a matter of debate.

Community Advisory Boards

As described previously, CABs, also called Community Advisory Groups, are formalized boards of individuals or stakeholder representatives that are intended to facilitate bidirectional communication between researchers, academic institutions, sponsors, and funders, on the one hand, and the community, on the other. Community representatives are identified through a range of strategies from self-selection of interested individuals to election to the CAB by community organizations or authorities.[23,37-38] These representatives engage with the researchers on a range of practical and ethical concerns such as understanding the potential risks and benefits of research, developing an appropriate consent process, and providing insight on community experiences of the research. Unlike participatory research processes, CAB members are not typically considered to be part of the research staff, and do not commonly participate in the trial procedures such as recruitment or data collection. Nevertheless, effective CABs require community representatives to be knowledgeable enough about the science to engage on issues arising in the research project. As a result, capacity building and training is an important part of CAB activities.[34,37-38] In addition, institutionally based CABs can address community concerns across a range of research projects at a research institution or clinical trial site[10,23] or across the activities of clinical trials units or networks.

Direct Engagement

Direct engagement refers to those methods of CE that prioritize the formation of direct relationships with diverse stakeholders in a community.[11,39-40] These engagement strategies tend to emphasize a consistent presence in the community through which researchers can build relationships with community members and capitalize on existing community institutions and processes to structure communication with the broader community. For example, a direct engagement strategy may emphasize communication with stakeholders through existing institutions and civil society groups such as town hall meetings, women's organizations, or religious institutions. In addition, they may involve outreach strategies into a community, such as targeted stakeholder meetings, focus group discussions, and surveys. In some circumstances, direct engagement is combined with CABs to expand the reach of engagement within the community.[11]

Forms of direct engagement have long been used in public health research, particularly in the global context.[37] For example, the Navrongo Health Research Centre in northern Ghana uses direct engagement with community leaders combined with conversations with the broader community about research activities through durbars, or traditional community gatherings.[41] Alternatively, in a community-based, vector-control research program in Mexico, the engagement strategy relied on the research team's consistent presence within the community. For instance, the principal investigator was in the town square every Saturday morning at the same time to talk with community members and discuss any concerns or questions in relation to the research.

Looking Ahead

The ethical importance of engaging communities in research has become increasingly well-recognized over the past twenty-five years. This awareness has translated into tangible changes in how research is conducted, particularly in HIV/AIDS research, and increasingly throughout biomedical research. These practices hold out great promise to improve the ethical quality of research by creating pathways through which to respond to the ethical dimensions of research, particularly as they have to do with justice in its conduct and outcomes. Nevertheless, serious obstacles remain in realizing this promise. Most notably, we do not have the evidence base necessary to determine what kinds of CE strategies are most effective in what research environments. As Peter Newman has argued, there is an urgent need to develop "a science of community engagement" that uses rigorous conceptual as well as empirical methods to better understand and evaluate methods of how best to engage with communities around research development, planning, and implementation.[42] The PCSBI[33] echoed this concern and recommended the development of evidence-based guidance to realize the promise of these practices both domestically and abroad.

When Is Community Engagement Required?

CE requires a significant investment of time, energy, and resources by a research program. Not every biomedical research study needs broad CE, but it is nearly certain that more studies should engage with communities than currently do. In this chapter, we considered a number of approaches to engagement with communities, from participatory research strategies in which communities are integrated into the knowledge production process as equal partners, to strategies that make use of CABs to structure and mediate relationships with the wider community. Even within these categories, there is significant diversity in objectives, intensity, and duration of the relationships, from programs that simply make stakeholders aware that certain research is going on and provide some opportunity for people to offer comments or submit questions, to engagement programs in which there are longstanding relationships between the research team and the stakeholder community, and which involve significant interaction, dialogue, and debate about the design and implementation of a research program.

Except for a limited number of circumstances, researchers have little guidance about what kind of engagement is required. Developing this guidance requires a better understanding of the theory and practice of CE. Theoretically, researchers need a clear articulation of the goals of CE, as well as with whom they have an obligation to engage.

The extreme view that researchers have an obligation to engage any and all groups with a legitimate interest does not seem plausible. But it is also not clear where to draw the line. That said, the interests-based approach to research community does point to a way forward. In particular, it is the extent to which research activities affect the interests of people, be they individuals or groups that trigger ethical obligations toward them. A reasonable starting place might be that the nature and extent of protections due to stakeholders corresponds to the extent to which their interests may be affected.

What Constitutes Meaningful Engagement?

Closely related to the question of when communities should be engaged is the question of what constitutes meaningful, or effective, engagement of those communities. Progress has been made in understanding the moral objectives of community engagement. A broad consensus about those goals is beginning to emerge, but more work remains to be done. In particular, these objectives need to be understood clearly and precisely enough that they can be operationalized in guidance for CE programs, and ultimately be used to evaluate the efficacy of those programs.

Take, for example, the goal of building legitimacy for a research program. Building legitimacy is widely discussed as an objective of meaningful CE programs, but it is not clear that CE, in its current forms, can achieve this objective. For example, many have questioned the representativeness of CABs, their accountability to the populations they claim to represent, and the grounds of their authority to represent often diffuse, unorganized populations.[34,38] In addition, there is a worry that CABs fail to legitimize research because they lack power to meaningfully influence the direction of research and so are little more than "window dressing."[33] In some cases, CABs are only formed after the key structural decisions about a trial have been made, leaving little opportunity for meaningful input into the design of the research.[39,43] In other instances, researchers may be unwilling to act on, or even consider, the input of the CABs on key decisions about the design or conduct of the trial.

In addition to understanding the goals of engagement, there is also a need for greater clarity about who makes up the research community, which the researcher has an obligation to engage. The concept of a research community is expansive, encompassing "stakeholders" to the research, or those groups and individuals who have a legitimate interest in the research. But, what makes an interest legitimate, and do researchers have a moral obligation to engage with all stakeholders who have this kind of legitimate interest?

Conclusion

Research ethics is undergoing a paradigm shift from a highly individualized ethics toward one that recognizes and accepts respecting communities as an obligation in biomedical research. CE, in all its diverse incarnations, aims to respond to this obligation by embedding research ethics within the complex social and political relationships that constitute a research community. Realizing the promise of CE, however, will also require a paradigm shift of a different sort. In particular, engaging communities effectively and efficiently will require a renewed emphasis on empirical research within human subjects protection. Historically, there has been a dearth of empirical data demonstrating the efficacy of human subjects' protections. CE, however, presents a unique and pressing opportunity to develop that strong empirical basis to ground regulations and guidance in this emerging area of human research protections.

Notes

1. Levine RJ. *Ethics and Regulation of Clinical Research*. Baltimore, MD: Yale University Press; 1988.
2. Streuwing JP, Abeliovich D, Peretz T, et. al. The carrier frequency of the BRCA1 185delAG mutation is approximately 1% in Ashkenazi Jewish individuals. *Nature Genetics*. 1995;11(2):198–200.
3. Levine RJ. Ashkenazi signals are timely. *Nature*. 1997;389(6649):315.
4. Genetic Information Nondiscrimination Act of 2008. 42 USC § 2000ff. Effective November 21, 2009.
5. Page-Shafer K, Saphonn V, Sun LP, Vun MC, Cooper DA, Kaldor JM. HIV prevention research in a resource-limited setting: the experience of planning a trial in Cambodia. *Lancet*. 2005;366(9495):1499–1503.
6. Global Campaign for Microbicides. *Preventing Prevention Trial Failures: A Case Study and Lessons for Future Trials from the 2004 Tenofovir Trial in Cambodia*. Washington, DC: Global Campaign for Microbicides at Program for Appropriate Technology in Health; 2009. http://www.global-campaign.org/clientfiles/Cambodia.pdf. Accessed December 4, 2017.
7. Ukpong M, Peterson K; New HIV Vaccine and Microbicide Advocacy Society. *Oral Tenofovir Controversy II : Voices from the Field*. Lagos, Nigeria: New HIV Vaccine and Microbicide Advocacy Society; 2009. http://www.nhvmas-ng.org/publication/TDF2.pdf. Accessed December 4, 2017.
8. Loff B, Jenkins C, Ditmore M, Overs C, Barbero R. Unethical clinical trials in Thailand: a community response. *Lancet*. 2005;365(9471):1618–1619.
9. Cox LE, Rouff JR, Svendsen KH, Markowitz M, Abrams DL. Community advisory boards: their role in AIDS clinical trials. *Health & Social Work*. 1998;23(4):290–297.
10. Community Partners. *Recommendations for Community Engagement in HIV/AIDS Research*. Seattle, WA: Office of HIV/AIDS Network Coordination; 2014. https://www.hanc.info/cp/resources/Documents/Recommendations%202014%20FINAL%206-5-14%20rc.pdf. Accessed December 4, 2017.
11. Joint United Nations Programme on HIV/AIDS (UNAIDS); Global Advocacy for HIV Protection. *Good Participatory Practice: Guidelines for Biomedical HIV Prevention Trials*. 2nd ed. Geneva, Switzerland: UNAIDS; 2011. http://www.avac.org/resource/good-participatory-practice-guidelines-biomedical-hiv-prevention-trials-second-edition. Accessed December 4, 2017.
12. Critical Path to TB Drug Regimens Initiative; Global Advocacy for HIV Protection. *Good Participatory Practice: Guidelines for TB Drug Trials*. New York, NY: Critical Path to TB Drug Regimens; 2012. http://www.cptrinitiative.org/downloads/resources/GPP-TB%20Oct1%202012%20FINAL.pdf. Accessed December 4, 2017.
13. Presidential Commission for the Study of Bioethical Issues. *Moral Science: Protecting Participants in Human Subjects Research*. Washington, DC: US Government Printing Office; 2012. https://bioethicsarchive.georgetown.

edu/pcsbi/sites/default/files/Moral%20Science%20June%202012.pdf. Accessed December 4, 2017.

14. Indian Health Service. Indian health manual. Part 1 General; Chapter 7 Research Activities. https://www.ihs.gov/ihm/index.cfm?module=dsp_ihm_pc_p1c7. Published May 6, 1987. Accessed December 4, 2017.

15. Canadian Institutes of Health Research; Natural Sciences and Engineering Research Council of Canada; Social Sciences and Humanities Research Council of Canada. *Tri-Council Policy Statement: Ethical Conduct for Research Involving Humans.* Ottawa, Canada: Interagency Secretariat on Research Ethics; 2014. http://www.pre.ethics.gc.ca/pdf/eng/tcps2-2014/TCPS_2_FINAL_Web.pdf. Accessed December 4, 2017.

16. National Bioethics Advisory Commission. *Research Involving Human Biological Materials: Ethical Issues and Policy Guidance*; Vol. 1. Rockville, MD: National Bioethics Advisory Commission; 1999. https://bioethicsarchive.georgetown. edu/nbac/hbm.pdf. Accessed December 4, 2017.

17. Sharp RR, Foster MW. Involving study populations in the review of genetic research. *Journal of Law, Medicine & Ethics.* 2000;28(1):41–51.

18. Sharp RR, Foster MW. Grappling with groups: protecting collective interests in biomedical research. *Journal of Medicine & Philosophy.* 2007;32(4):321–337.

19. Simon CM, Newbury E, L'heureux J. Protecting participants, promoting progress: public perspectives on community advisory boards (CABs) in biobanking. *Journal of Empirical Research on Human Research Ethics.* 2011;6(3):19–30.

20. Lemke AA, Wolf WA, Hebert-Beirne JH, Smith ME. Public and biobank participant attitudes toward genetic research participation and data sharing. *Public Health Genomics.* 2010;13(6):368–377.

21. Clinical and Translational Science Awards Consortium's Community Engagement Key Function Committee Task Force. *Principles of Community Engagement.* 2nd ed. Bethesda, MD: National Institutes of Health; 2011. NIH publication 11-7782. https://www.atsdr.cdc.gov/communityengagement/pdf/ PCE_Report_508_FINAL.pdf. Accessed December 4, 2017.

22. Holzer J, Kass N. Community engagement strategies in the original and renewal applications for CTSA grant funding. *Clinical and Translational Science.* 2013;7(1):38–43.

23. Marsh V, Kamuya D, Rowa Y, Gikonyo C, Molyneux S. Beginning community engagement at a busy biomedical research programme: experiences from the KEMRI CGMRC-Wellcome Trust Research Programme, Kilifi, Kenya. *Social Science & Medicine.* 2008;67(5):721–733.

24. Dickert N, Sugarman J. Ethical goals of community consultation in research. *American Journal of Public Health.* 2005;95(7):1123–1127.

25. Joint United Nations Programme on HIV/AIDS (UNAIDS); World Health Organization (WHO). *Ethical Considerations in Biomedical HIV Prevention Trials: UNAIDS/WHO Guidance Document.* Geneva, Switzerland: UNAIDS;

2012. http://www.unaids.org/sites/default/files/media_asset/jc1399_ethical_considerations_en_0.pdf. Accessed December 4, 2017.

26. King KF, Kolopack P, Merritt MW, Lavery JV. Community engagement and the human infrastructure of global health research. *BMC Medical Ethics.* 2014;15(1):84.

27. Mello MM, Wolf LE. The Havasupai Indian tribe case–lessons for research involving stored biologic samples. *New England Journal of Medicine.* 2010;363(3):201–204.

28. Darwall SL. Two kinds of respect. *Ethics.* 1977;88(1):36–49.

29. Frankfurt H. Equality and respect. *Social Research.* 1997;64(1):3–15.

30. Raz J. *Value, Respect, and Attachment.* Cambridge, England: Cambridge University Press; 2001.

31. Dickert NW. Re-examining respect for human research participants. *Kennedy Institute of Ethics Journal.* 2009;19(4):311–338.

32. Emanuel EJ, Wendler D, Killen J, Grady C. What makes clinical research in developing countries ethical? The benchmarks of ethical research. *Journal of Infectious Diseases.* 2011;189(1):930–937.

33. Presidential Commission for the Study of Bioethical Issues. *Research Across Borders: Proceedings of the International Research Panel of the Presidential Commission for the Study of Bioethical Issues.* Washington, DC: US Government Printing Office; 2011. https://bioethicsarchive.georgetown.edu/pcsbi/sites/default/files/IRP-%20Research%20Across%20Borders.pdf. Accessed December 4, 2017.

34. Weijer C, Goldsand G, Emanuel EJ. Protecting communities in research: current guidelines and limits of extrapolation. *Nature Genetics.* 1999;23(3):275–280.

35. Cargo M, Mercer SL. The value and challenges of participatory research: strengthening its practice. *Annual Review of Public Health.* 2008;29(1):325–350.

36. Israel BA, Coombe CM, Cheezum RR, et al. Community-based participatory research: a capacity-building approach for policy advocacy aimed at eliminating health disparities. *American Journal of Public Health.* 2010;100(11):2094–2102.

37. Kamuya DM, Marsh V, Kombe FK, Geissler PW, Molyneux SC. Engaging communities to strengthen research ethics in low-income settings: selection and perceptions of members of a network of representatives in Coastal Kenya. *Developing World Bioethics.* 2013;13(1):10–20.

38. Shubis K, Juma O, Sharifu R, Burgess B, Abdulla S. Challenges of establishing a Community Advisory Board (CAB) in a low-income, low-resource setting: experiences from Bagamoyo, Tanzania. *Health Research Policy and Systems.* 2009;7:16.

39. Tindana PO, Singh JA, Tracy CS, et al. Grand challenges in global health: community engagement in research in developing countries. *PLoS Medicine.* 2007;4(9):e273.
40. Lavery JV, Tindana PO, Scott TW, et al. Towards a framework for community engagement in global health research. *Trends Parasitology.* 2010;26(6):279–283.
41. Tindana PO, Rozmovits L, Boulanger RF, et al. Aligning community engagement with traditional authority structures in global health research: a case study from Northern Ghana. *American Journal of Public Health.* 2011;101(10):1857–1867.
42. Newman PA. Towards a science of community engagement. *Lancet.* 2006;367(9507):302.
43. Quinn SC. Protecting human subjects: the role of community advisory boards. *American Journal of Public Health.* 2004;94(6):918–922.

9 JUSTICE AND RESEARCH WITH CONVENIENT AND CAPTIVE POPULATIONS

Jonathan D. Moreno*

A subject population that is convenient is one that is easily accessible and available for recruitment or for monitoring through the course of a study. This chapter will examine three examples of such identifiable populations: prisoners, military personnel, and those in "status relationships" (those of lesser power) such as students and research staff.

Some of these individuals are convenient in the sense that they are readily available, such as students. Others are not only readily available but also captive, that is, constrained in their movements and choices by virtue of explicit conditions formally imposed on them by societal decision. The paradigm case of a captive population is those who are imprisoned. Other populations seem to occupy a middle ground between short-term hospitalized patients and long-term prisoners, and include students and military personnel. Among the ways that these populations differ from other potential subject populations are their degree of availability and the greater likelihood that those who are captive can be coerced or manipulated into participation by virtue of their dependent status. Also, captive populations are more likely than others to be readily available for research activities for extended periods, enhancing their attractiveness to the research enterprise (e.g., by potentially minimizing research costs as well as controlling for variability in the research environment to improve data quality).

The growing sensitivity to the use of such populations in research cannot be understood without an appreciation of the

* The author expresses his gratitude to Kate Odululkwe for her assistance in the preparation of the manuscript.

historical background. The history of research on these subject populations is important because it provides the rationale for classifying them as "vulnerable." The discussion of each particular subject population also includes an account of the way the regulatory system has evolved to take account of historic abuses.

Because these groups are not convenient or captive—or even vulnerable—in the same ways, crafting a just, efficacious, and reasonable public policy in the use of these populations in biomedical and behavioral research is not easy. For instance, a rough notion of justice may find it acceptable to impose greater burdens on prisoners because of their debt to society. Similarly, it might be argued that those who are institutionalized, such as prisoners, may need to be used to serve some important research goal, especially if no other population so readily presents itself for study. Nevertheless, historically, these attitudes have sometimes had baleful consequences. Further, our intuitions about justice in research may yield inconsistent results. For example, turning soldiers into "guinea pigs" may either be offensive to patriotic sensibilities or seem reasonable in light of martial duties. Students and laboratory workers could be viewed either as too easily influenced to participate in research or as the most appropriate candidates due to their ability to understand an experiment's purposes.

All these views have been represented in the history of biomedical research with these populations, indicating how important it has been to craft a coherent and historically informed conception of justice in research, forged to fit the special nature of convenient and captive populations. One element that crops up repeatedly in the research context, for which a more general notion of justice is ill-prepared, is that human subjects are often used in research that is not intended to benefit them, but instead to benefit other individuals. Likewise, a population may be used in studies that develop treatments intended mainly, or exclusively, to benefit other groups. To be reasonable, suitable, and practical, any reasonably well-formed conception of justice in research will need to reckon with these special circumstances.

While discussions such as this tend to focus on ethical abuses or areas of potential moral concern, it should be remembered, however, that much human-subject research has contributed greatly to human well-being and has been conducted according to sound ethical standards. Such standards include efforts to prevent the burdens of research from falling unfairly on any particular person or group. This chapter will show how attitudes toward certain populations from which research subjects may be drawn have changed, and to indicate that some of the issues remain to be resolved.

This chapter's focus on convenient or captive populations is limited to examination of justice issues arising in research with prisoners, military personnel, and those in "status relationships" such as students and research staff. The use of hospitalized patients in research and institutionalized patients with cognitive disabilities, although falling within the category of convenient or captive populations, will not be discussed because they are covered in detail in Chapters 3 and 4, respectively, of this volume. Another sort of readily available, captive population is exemplified by the African American men who were subject to the so-called Tuskegee Syphilis Study, better named the United States Public Health Service Syphilis Study, discussed in Chapter 7 in this volume. These men were available and convenient by virtue of their social status. Yet another example is that of the Navajo uranium miners and millers, who were observed for the carcinogenic results of their occupation for years, also by the US Public Health Service. Observational studies arising from conditions that have not been created by investigators, but arise in nature, are also called "experiments of opportunity."[1]

Justice Over Time

Prisoners

There is no population more fully captive than the long-term prisoner. Among the apocrypha of medical history are tales of the use of living criminals as subjects in various medical studies in the ancient world, including poison experiments and vivisection. In the eighteenth century European physicians exposed prisoners to sexually transmitted infections (STIs), cancers, typhoid, and scarlet fever. An influential study of pellagra in 1914 used Mississippi convicts and presaged greater use of this population.[2] During World War II in the United States many prisoners participated in studies of conditions such as malaria and STIs.

After the war, a trial of those accused of conducting horrific experiments on concentration camp inmates was held in Nuremberg, Germany. The defense attorneys in the trial pointed to cases of prison research in the United States and elsewhere as part of their justification for their clients' conduct. Among the many instances cited by the Nazis' lawyers were the pellagra and malaria studies, as well as that of an American team of researchers who received permission from the governor of the Philippines to use condemned criminals and other convicts in typhus and beriberi experiments.[3]

Although the Nuremberg judges sentenced some of the defendants to death and others to lengthy jail sentences for experiments on concentration camp prisoners, there was little apparent effect on the conduct of research involving American prisoners. During the war American prisoners were known as and considered to be "volunteers," while the victims of Nazi experiments were seen as forced participants. In fact, at the same time that Illinois physician Andrew Ivy was authoring portions of what would become the Nuremberg Code (as the American Medical Association's representative at the trial), he also chaired a committee appointed by the governor of Illinois to review the ethics of prison research. The committee argued for constraints on the use of prisoners in research but implicitly endorsed the continued use of this population. Reporting only a few months after the Nazi doctors' trial, Ivy's committee effectively forestalled the direct application of the results of the trial to American prison research.[4] Several years later, an early draft of the Declaration of Helsinki that would have explicitly prohibited prison research was revised at US insistence.[5]

Over the next decade several drug manufacturers made substantial investments in prison research, and in some cases erected buildings with state-of-the-art laboratory facilities at penitentiaries. By 1960, as many as 20,000 federal prisoners were participants in medical experiments.[6] In 1973 the Pharmaceutical Manufacturers Association estimated that about 70 percent of Phase I drug tests were carried out on prisoners, or about 3,600 individuals.[7] American prisoners and prison-based facilities were also being used to test drugs for sponsors abroad.[7]

Some prison experiments were sponsored by the federal government. One involved the irradiation of the testicles of 131 prisoners in state penitentiaries in Oregon and Washington State between 1963 and 1973, and was funded by the Atomic Energy Commission (AEC). There were clear rules in place within the AEC that should have applied to these studies, including a requirement for written consent from subjects. However, in 1995 the President's Advisory Committee on Human Radiation Experiments found that these rules were not fully observed in the testicular irradiation research.[1]

Among the attractions to research for prisoners were far higher pay than afforded by other prison jobs, the possibility of a more favorable parole status, a break in the boredom of incarceration, and often better food and living conditions. A 1974 editorial in the *Journal of Legal Medicine* argued that as long as prisoners are free to enter and leave a research program at any time, and if they understand the hazards of participation, they should be free to make this choice. The writer suggested that it would be "immoral in itself to deny them this opportunity," and "an abridgment of whatever civil and constitutional rights they may possess" (p. 6).[8] So it was argued that their very rehabilitation could turn on this decision. "There is no doubt," the editorial concluded, "that biomedical research is an absolute necessity if society is to survive" (p. 6).[8] Implicit in this conclusion was that prisoners are a critically important subject pool in the advancement of science.

In the mid-1970s the use of prison inmates in medical research in the United States began to decline sharply, and was finally reduced almost to the point of extinction. One reason for the change in practice was a recommendation by the US National Commission for the Protection of Human Subjects of Biomedical and Behavioral Research (National Commission) in 1976 that a moratorium be declared on prisoner experiments pending the adoption of some minimum standards. The Commission's recommendation followed a notorious and bloody prison riot at the Attica State Penitentiary (Attica) in September 1971. The Attica disturbances met with a fierce response by New York State Police that left dozens of African American prisoners dead and exposed the awful living conditions to which the prisoners had been subjected. Attica cast a novel and unflattering light on the coercive nature of prison life, and, to many, the coercive nature of using prisoners in research.[4] The commission's moratorium proposal met with fierce criticism from virtually every affected party—physicians, advocates, and the prisoners themselves. One distinguished commentator, Louis Lasagna, charged that the National Commission's recommendations "illustrate beautifully how well-intentioned desires to protect prisoners can lead otherwise intelligent people to destroy properly performed research that scrupulously involves informed consent and full explanation and avoids coercion to the satisfaction of all but the most tunnel-visioned doctrinaire" (p. 2349).[9] The US DHEW (Department of Health, Education, and Welfare, a predecessor to the US Department of Health and Human Services) instead promulgated regulations that effectively prohibited nearly all prison research.

The premise that prison research is acceptable if prisoners are free to decline to participate is, admittedly, question-begging, and the proposition that society's survival depends on biomedical research is, if not hyperbolic, in need of defense. On the other hand, there may be validity in the claim that research participation can forge a sense of connection to society among those who otherwise have little opportunity to feel part of any community beyond the institution. As the National Commission heard from one inmate, "It makes a prisoner feel good to volunteer. It makes him feel like he's doing something productive."[10] On the other hand, the primary reason the National Commission heard for volunteering was financial, since opportunities in prison to earn money for oneself or loved ones on the outside are few.[10]

Currently prison research is allowable under federal regulations for only four highly restricted kinds of research: minimal risk research on incarceration and criminal behavior, studies of prisons as institutions or prisoners as incarcerated persons, research on conditions that particularly affect prisoners as a class, and studies of therapies likely to benefit the prisoner.[11] Under the last two conditions prison studies have been conducted on multidrug–resistant tuberculosis, a disease common in prisons due to the combination of density of living conditions and a high prevalence of HIV.[12]

There has, therefore, been a shift from well-established use of prisoners for research purposes to a protectionist regulatory scheme. To find a proposed research project ethically sound, this protectionist philosophy requires a narrow construal of potential benefits to prisoners as a group or as individuals. There is considerable irony about the formation of the current public policy concerning prison research. In the most thorough scholarly analysis of the policy shift that took place in the late 1970s on the use of prisoners as subjects, historian Jon Harkness concludes that there was no contemporary social consensus on the matter. Instead, Harkness contends, retrospective consensus formed in opposition to prison research only after it had been banned by DHEW for judicial, rather than ethical, reasons.[4]

A widespread moral intuition that prison research is inherently untenable from an ethical standpoint seems to have come about without benefit of information about the facts of the practice in question. For example, one might suppose that prison research invites exploitation of inmates, persons who are often among the most vulnerable groups in our society. But it is well documented that for most of the post–World War II period African American prisoners were, if anything, underrepresented as prison research subjects. The reason for this was that participation in medical experiments was considered to be a privilege that would be afforded mainly to white convicts. This situation only began to change with the success of the civil rights movement.[4] Similarly, as noted by a leading medical ethicist (Robert J. Levine, MD, oral communication, April 1997), by the 1960s untoward inducements for prisoner participation in research, such as time granted toward parole and high reimbursement rates, were being significantly curtailed. All this suggests that, if the potential for coercion is taken to be the main problem of prisoners' research participation, it may not have formed a credible basis for the ultimate strict curtailment of their inclusion.

However, such a line of analysis presupposes that coercion is the only ethical problem with prison research. According to the ethical principles articulated by the National Commission in its *Belmont Report* (respect for persons, beneficence, and justice), prison research would create ethical difficulties even if conducted in a manner consistent with respect for persons and beneficence because it singles out a specific population for research participation, which will then be disproportionate in numbers to that of other groups.[13]

Thus, even if the problem of coercion was resolved to our complete satisfaction, and even if we knew that research participation advances the rehabilitation process, enrolling prisoners in research would still be problematic. Since prisoners have in fact played a disproportionate role in research whenever and wherever such research has been permitted, their use would normally be unethical no matter how ethically satisfactory the research was in other respects.

This objection would not apply in cases in which the medical or behavioral problem to be studied occurs disproportionately in the prison population, consistent with both the letter and the spirit of the current US federal regulations governing prison research. Recognizing that in many respects the prison population suffers not because of the exploitation of medical and behavioral research but because of a lack of knowledge of the unique problems facing prisoners, in 2006 the US Institute of Medicine (IOM, now known as the National Academy of Medicine) recommended reforms in the conduct of research in prisons. The IOM committee (of which the author was a member) observed that vast changes had taken place in the nature of the prison population and in their conditions since the *Belmont Report* and the subsequent federal regulations, including a more than 4.5-fold increase in the number of prisoners, greater overcrowding of correctional facilities, and the confinement of more disadvantaged populations than was the case in the 1970s. Furthermore, it was noted that, for certain studies, IRBs might require that the proportion of prisoner-subjects to nonprisoner-subjects may not exceed 50 percent, thus addressing historical concerns about overrepresentation and minimizing the likelihood that prisoners could be singled out for especially risky research.[14]

Military Personnel

Military personnel are convenient subjects in the sense that they are typically healthy, "normal" persons who can be followed for data collection for a number of years. However, their disciplined environment raises questions about the extent to which any consent they give can be considered truly voluntary. They thus may be at risk for disproportionate representation in research, especially in studies relating to national security. Yet military officials have long considered voluntariness an important condition for participation in research by military personnel, as evidenced by the use of the term "volunteer" or "informed volunteer" from at least the 1940s (pp. 45–73).[1] The precise significance to be given the term under the circumstances is, of course, a separate but vitally important matter.

The American record in the use of military personnel in research has been mixed. In some cases truly pioneering policies have been inconsistently applied, undermining their force. Around 1900, US Army scientist Walter Reed obtained consent and asked potential subjects to sign a written contract for his yellow fever experiment in Cuba. The contract specified some of the risks, and offered monetary compensation to participants, perhaps high enough to be considered undue influence today. There was also little opportunity to withdraw from the study.

Though Reed began his dangerous experiment without his superior's approval, he felt obliged to ask his commanding officer's permission when he thought it necessary to expand the study. Since at least the 1930s it appears that approval for soldiers' and sailors' participation in medical experiments was to be obtained at the highest level of the relevant uniformed service, usually from the appropriate service surgeon general and often the service secretary as well. The assignment of military personnel to research is, after all, a deployment decision that should theoretically be made by the responsible officer in the chain of command.

There are also significant potential risks to the armed forces if an experiment goes awry, especially in terms of public opinion and legal liability, constituting another reason for proper authorization of human research. During World War II the White House's Committee on Medical Research declared that uniformed personnel were not to be used as "guinea pigs" in the war-related research it funded. Throughout this period there was significant concern that the public would not be sympathetic if their heroes were to be used in this manner. Nonetheless, during the war naval personnel were forced to remain in mustard gas experiments against their will.[15]

By the late 1940s there was a growing view in the national security establishment that some human experiments were going to be necessary in the post-war environment, especially in reference to unconventional weapons, atomic, biological, and chemical. The effects of these weapons could not be gauged in animal studies, nor could their combat implications be assessed with other healthy subjects. Early 1950s studies of flash-blindness following atomic detonations, for example, were classified by the Pentagon as medical experiments, though most other exposures to the atomic battlefield were considered to be part of needed training.[15] The US Department of Defense attempted to anticipate the problem of using military personnel in research by adopting the Nuremberg Code as its policy in 1953. Subsequently, troops deployed near the site of atomic tests were systematically observed and sometimes filed self-reports of panic reactions near the blast site. "Release" forms were even filled out in at least some cases by troops who had "volunteered" to operate closer to ground zero than others, thus exposing them to a higher level of radioactivity. Yet in other studies involving military personnel and radiation there was no documentation of volunteer status except the statements of superior officers.[15] In still other cases, such as the US air force's mushroom-cloud–penetration experiments that measured the amount of fission released by an atomic blast and its effects on crew members, there is strong evidence that at least some Air Force personnel were eager to experience the challenge and adventure associated with the project, while others viewed it as part of their routine.[15]

The military context presents a unique puzzle about distinguishing training, which does not typically fall under the constraints of medical ethics, from medical research, which does. For instance, the vast majority of the "atomic soldiers" deployed for exercises at the training facility at Camp Desert Rock in Nevada from 1951 to 1962 were kept at what was thought to be a safe distance from the atomic blast site; though any acute ill-effects might have been noted, the primary goal of the activity was to learn about human factors such as panic reactions on the atomic battlefield. Although the tension between national security needs and ethical considerations was rarely a topic of public discussion during the Cold War, it played an important role in shaping the defense establishment's ambivalent posture toward human subjects issues.[15]

The implementation of the Nuremberg Code–based policy appears to have been sporadic at best, perhaps partly because there was confusion about its scope and application. The US Army Inspector General found in 1975 that the Army had failed to comply with its own rules for the use of soldiers in research with psychoactive drugs, as thousands of soldiers were used in LSD experiments in the 1950s.[16] Even in the courts the code has not proven to be an effective standard. When one of the men brought suit against the United States government for injuries he incurred due to this research, the US Supreme Court ruled in favor of the government by a five-to-four majority on the grounds that the judicial branch should not undermine discipline by inquiring into military matters. Only the minority argued that the Nuremberg Code must prevail.[17]

Policies have been adopted to bring military research practices into compliance with practices in civilian settings. In 1991 the US Department of Defense regulations on the use of human subjects were brought under the same requirements as other federal agencies that sponsor studies with human subjects.[18] There are additional regulatory obstacles limiting recruitment of military personnel for research so that today this is among the most difficult populations from which to obtain subjects. Today, all research in the Army's infectious disease institute at Fort Detrick, for example, is governed by several regulations and all proposals involving significant risk must be reviewed by a local IRB, the Human Use Review and Regulatory Affairs Division of the United States Army Medical Research and Material Command, the Human Subjects Research Review Board of the Office of the Surgeon General, and the Office of the Surgeon General itself.[19] In response to the recommendations of the Advisory Committee on Human Radiation Experiments, in 1997 President William J. Clinton ordered expanded training for senior officers on the nature of human subjects research, and instituted a new policy that precludes officers from involvement in the recruitment of research volunteers.[20]

Other events illustrate the special ethical difficulties associated with regulating the use of innovative drugs with military personnel during a national emergency. In late 1990 and early 1991, during Operations Desert Shield and Desert Storm, the US Defense Department was concerned about possible exposure to biological and chemical warfare agents. The department successfully sought an amendment to the US Food and Drug Administration's informed consent regulations that would enable medical professionals to determine that it was "not feasible" to obtain the informed consent of a person receiving an investigational drug or vaccine under combat conditions. The rule was published on December 21, 1990, and upheld by the courts.[21]

Shortly after the rule was published the US Department of Defense requested and received waivers of informed consent for two investigational products: pyridostigmine bromide (PB) and botulinum toxoid (BT). It should be noted that PB was an anti–myasthenia gravis drug intended to protect against chemical weapons, and that the BT drug was to be used as a protective measure from prepoisonous botulinum toxins.[22] Even though the waiver was obtained for both agents, Central Command elected on ethical grounds to give service personnel a choice about receiving BT, but not for PB, which was in common use as an approved drug for other populations and for which informed consent was not deemed necessary. The Pentagon estimates that about 8,000 troops took BT and about 250,000 received at least one dose of PB.[22]

Months after the war some veterans began complaining about numerous symptoms that when grouped together are termed "Gulf War Syndrome." The vaccination program was shrouded in secrecy when it took place to deny information to the enemy about the allies' defensive measures, but as the story emerged the agents, especially PB, were theorized by some as a factor in the veterans' medical problems. A federal advisory committee was appointed to investigate the health problems of Gulf War veterans, including an analysis of the waiver process.[22] It can be argued that use of agents that have not yet been approved for use under ordinary circumstances may be ethical during combat. The lack of approval could be due to technical or bureaucratic factors and there may be sound scientific evidence that the agent can be of significant potential benefit to troops in combat.[23]

Underlying much of the criticism of the Defense Department's conduct in the use of unapproved agents is a suspicion that it was a deliberate effort to circumvent research requirements in order to assess the agents' efficacy under combat conditions. There is no evidence that this is the case. Indeed, one shortcoming of the department's handling of this episode is precisely the fact that no system was in place to document the response of service personnel to the medications, including a failure to establish appropriate baseline measures of subjects' metabolism.[24] The use of these compounds "in theater" could theoretically have been justified on scientific as well as beneficent grounds if the operation had been treated as a research study according to established methodological standards.

Had a systematic research dimension been part of the agents' use in Desert Storm, there would then have been an opportunity to assess the fairness of conducting research with military personnel. The assessment would have turned on the manner in which the study was conducted, for while soldiers facing combat conditions may be required to accept all medical interventions that hold the prospect of ensuring their availability for service, the innovative use of these agents may not entail a requirement to accept them. On the other hand, if the decision to use the agents could have been left to the troops themselves, with appropriate information at their disposal about known risks and benefits, then their study participation would have been acceptable. Apparently this information about the risks and benefits was not made available in Desert Storm, in spite of an agreement between the Defense Department and the Food and Drug Administration that it would be provided.[25]

Students

Students are captive in a different sense from any of the groups mentioned thus far. They exemplify persons who are in a social context characterized by power relations. In particular, their differential role is characterized by inherently lesser power than the other member of the relationship, in this instance a teacher. Students are by no means unique in this sense; other relationships that are characterized by power differentials are employers and employees, and supervisors and laboratory workers. In general, whatever recruitment policies are established for students in research might reasonably apply to those who are similarly vulnerable by virtue of other power relationships.

A college or graduate student may face a course requirement that they serve as a study subject or write a paper, an unattractive alternative for many busy students. Or they may respond to campus or local advertisements offering cash in exchange for volunteering for research. As these students are often unemployed or underemployed, even small monetary inducements can be influential in their decision-making about research participation. Perhaps because the kind of research to which students are usually subjected is behavioral and presents minimal physical risk (though arguably sometimes psychological risk), and there has been no great scandal about participation in studies as a course requirement, this population had long received the least attention among those who may be said to be in an environment that involves undue influence to participate in research.

In one sense college and graduate students are close to ideal candidates because of their potential intellectual identification with the research; the only superior subjects in this sense are the researchers themselves.[26] The creation of special obstacles to the enrollment of these students, who are generally regarded as the "best and the brightest" by their faculties and far less likely to be exploited than other societal groups, may be viewed as institutional paternalism.[27] Nevertheless, there is evidence that medical students do not believe their professors' consent processes are adequate.[28] In an attempt to address lingering concerns about student research participation the American Psychological Association's code of ethics provides that, "When psychologists conduct research with clients/patients, students or subordinates as participants, psychologists take steps to protect the prospective participants from adverse consequences of declining or withdrawing from participation," and that, "When research participation is a course requirement or an opportunity for extra credit, the prospective participant is given the choice of equitable alternative activities" (p. 10).[29]

Finally, there is again the issue of financial compensation. The American Psychological Association requires that, "Psychologists make reasonable efforts to avoid offering excessive or inappropriate financial or other inducements for research participation when such inducements are likely to coerce participation" (p. 11).[29] In order to avoid asserting undue influence, remuneration for study participation should take into account the financial position of the population from which subjects are to be recruited. Many students live on loans that present them with a significant burden for many years. Compensation may take into account expenses associated with study participation, such as travel. Additional amounts should be calculated based on a reasonable assessment of the value of the time invested by members of that population. Thus, for example, asserting undue influence would be offering a hundred dollars an hour to an individual who could not otherwise earn a fraction of that amount. This example applies to more groups than students, of course, including persons in the developing world.

Spanning Populations: The Guatemala Studies

A somewhat recently disclosed incident is both relevant to several captive and convenient populations and introduces an international dimension (see also Chapter 10). This particularly egregious series of studies that was conducted by the United States government in mid-twentieth-century Guatemala only came to light in 2010. In a post–World War II effort primarily to determine whether penicillin is an effective postexposure treatment for sexually transmitted infections, the Guatemala experiments involved prisoners, institutionalized persons (mental patients and Hansen disease patients), and soldiers. The project appears to have been motivated partly by the significant STI burden on American military personnel during World War II. The research that took place mainly from July 1946 to December 1948 was a collaborative effort of the Pan American Sanitary Bureau (now the Pan American Health Organization), the US Public Health Service Venereal Disease Research Laboratory, and various authorities in the Guatemalan government and institutions. The international and intergovernmental aspect of the experiments gives the Guatemala case a distinct character from others discussed in this chapter.

The key methodology of the Guatemala experiments was intentional exposure of 1,308 persons to syphilis, gonorrhea, or chancroid, accomplished through sexual exposure, superficial inoculation into the penis, deep inoculation into the penis, and superficial inoculation following sexual exposure. There were also inoculations in the rectum, urethra, and/or eyes. Testing for new diagnostic techniques continued through 1953, including blood draws and lumbar punctures. Commercial sex workers and at least one child soldier were also involved in some phases of the experiments.

Following the public revelation of the experiments by historian Susan Reverby, US President Barack Obama issued an official apology to the president of Guatemala in 2010. US Secretary of State Hillary Clinton and Health and Human Services Secretary Kathleen Sebelius also apologized to the government of Guatemala and both the survivors and descendants of those infected.[30] Subsequently, the administration charged the US Presidential Commission for the Study of Bioethical Issues with investigating the facts and circumstances of the experiments. In its 2011 report, the commission found that, by the ethical standards of that time and without imposing retrospective ethical conventions, "many of the actions of the researchers were morally wrong and the individual researchers and institutional officials were morally blameworthy" (p. 9).[31]

Looking Ahead

Because they are captive in very different ways, justice in research with the noted subject populations must be assessed quite differently. For instance, the ready availability of institutionalized persons like prisoners would seem to make them prime research candidates, especially considering the prevalence of mental illness, a history of drug use, and other behavioral problems in that population. However, prison research is far from a flourishing enterprise, owing both to regulatory constraints and a lack of funding. Further, aspects of current prison settings are not conducive to research. For example, research on mental illness would likely require identifying prisoners with severe mental illness and placing them in facilities where they can receive adequate psychiatric care.

Similarly, military personnel are not likely to be involved in the pursuit of generalizable knowledge in the foreseeable future. In general, for both political and moral reasons there has been an historic reluctance to use military personnel in research when others are available. Today, somewhat more plausible than explicitly pressing soldiers into such service as research subjects (concerning which there are considerable bureaucratic and political hurdles) could be *de facto* field testing of a new drug or procedure under conditions of armed conflict. This applies especially when the drug or procedure has a track record of safety and efficacy in previous studies. Innovative neurotechnologies include devices that are of interest to military planners. One example could be the deployment of transcranial magnetic stimulation devices believed by some to be capable of enhancing attention and cognition.[32] That scenario treats the activity as "program evaluation" or "quality assessment" rather than research, which may amount to a thin evasion of the research rules.

In other respects, considering how much use is made of young people like students in medical and behavioral research, even a few isolated tragedies could excite considerable public alarm. Some further restrictions on the use of students in research seem likely, at least at local levels, perhaps by prohibiting their recruitment by their current instructors.

In 2017, the US federal government issued new regulations to reform the current research review system. Those regulations, scheduled to be effective in 2018, calibrate the level of review to the level of risk entailed by the study.[33] One result of this revision might be that behavioral studies of the prison environment will require less review than is currently the case (so long as issues like privacy of sensitive information like drug use and sexual activity are addressed by a proposed new data security system). Similar calibrated adjustments could be made for research involving military personnel and students. However, it will take time and experience as the new framework is implemented to understand its impact on how justice in research will be assured for convenient and captive populations.

Conclusion

In crafting a just public policy for the use of human subjects, especially those who may be considered convenient or captive, the historical and practical factors that could enter into judgments about justice will vary depending on what population is being considered and that population's particular circumstances. The respective situations of prisoners, military personnel, and students are quite different and require analyses tailored to each group. Underlying all these cases are complex issues of social status and power, as well as medical ethics.

As experience in modern research with human subjects has accumulated, a "protectionist" attitude toward the participation of these groups has emerged. However, a protectionist stance toward certain populations does not rule out the possibility that strong arguments for research participation can be mounted. Surely there are circumstances in which justice may permit, or even require, access to research for populations that have historically been abused by researchers. One of these circumstances is the prevalence of a condition that poses a particular threat to members of that population, and which cannot be studied as effectively with other subjects. Protected status implies institutional and public scrutiny of proposed research participation, not a priori exclusion. With this understanding, and in light of the historical factors that have made these groups' participation in biomedical and behavioral research a matter of special concern, protectionism continues to be a morally sound presumption for them.

Notes

1. Advisory Committee on Human Radiation Experiments. *The Human Radiation Experiments: Final Report of the President's Advisory Committee.* New York, NY: Oxford University Press; 1996.
2. Etheridge EW. *The Butterfly Caste: A Social History of Pellagra in the South.* Westport, CT: Greenwood Publishing Company; 1972.
3. *Trials of War Criminals Before the Nuernberg Military Tribunals Under Control Council Law No. 10; Nuernberg, October 1946–April 1949.* Washington,

DC: US Government Printing Office; 1950. https://archive.org/stream/trialsofwarcrimi06inte/trialsofwarcrimi06inte_djvu. Accessed October 28, 2016.

4. Harkness JM. *Research Behind Bars: A History of Nontherapeutic Research on American Prisoners* [dissertation]. Madison: University of Wisconsin; 1996.

5. National Commission for the Protection of Human Subjects of Biomedical and Behavioral Research. *Research Involving Prisoners: Appendix to Report and Recommendations.* Washington, DC: US Government Printing Office; 1976.

6. Fox RC. *Experiment Perilous: Physicians and Patients Facing the Unknown.* New Brunswick, NJ: Transaction Publishers; 1997.

7. Our Washington correspondent. Prison research: ethics behind bars. *Nature.* 1973;242(5394):153.

8. Trout ME. Should research in prisons be barred? *Journal of Legal Medicine (N Y).* 1974;2(5):6.

9. Lasagna L. Prisoner subjects and drug testing. *Federation Proceedings.* 1977;36(10):2349–2351.

10. Cohn V. Inmates oppose experiment halt. *Washington Post.* November 16, 1975:A1+.

11. US Department of Health and Human Services. Protection of human subjects: additional protections pertaining to biomedical and behavioral research involving prisoners as subjects. 45 CFR §46, subpart C. http://www.hhs.gov/ohrp/regulations-and-policy/regulations/45-cfr-46/#. Revised January 15, 2009. Effective July 14, 2009. Accessed December 4, 2017.

12. Potler C, Sharp VL, Remick S. Prisoners' access to HIV experimental trials: legal, ethical, and practical considerations. *Journal of Acquired Immune Deficiency Syndromes.* 1994;7(10):1086–1094.

13. National Commission for the Protection of Human Subjects of Biomedical and Behavioral Research. The Belmont Report: Ethical principles and guidelines for the protection of human subjects of research. *Federal Register.* 1979;44(76):23192–23197.

14. Gostin LO, Vanchieri C, Pope A, eds. *Ethical Considerations for Research Involving Prisoners.* Washington, DC: National Academies Press; 2007.

15. Pechura CM, Rall DP, eds. *Veterans at Risk: The Health Effects of Mustard Gas and Lewisite.* Washington, DC: National Academy Press; 1993.

16. Downey TJ. Report on human experimentation conducted or funded by the U.S. Army. *Congressional Record.* 1975;121(130):H8446-H8450.

17. *United States v. Stanley,* 483 U.S. 669 (1987).

18. US Department of Health and Human Services. Federal policy for the protection of human subjects; notices and rules. *Federal Register.* 1991;56(117):28002–28032.

19. US Army Medical Research Institute of Infectious Disease. *USAMRIID 70-25, 4.b: Use of Human Subjects in Research.* Washington, DC: US Department of the Army; 1995.

20. Human Radiation Interagency Working Group. *Building Public Trust: Actions to Respond to the Report of the Advisory Committee on Human Radiation Experiments.* Washington, DC: US Department of Energy; 1997.

21. Presidential Advisory Committee on Gulf War Veterans' Illnesses. *Interim Report*. Washington, DC: US Government Printing Office; 1996.

22. Roberts J. Debate over U.S. Gulf war syndrome continues. *BMJ*. 1994;309(6966):1392-1393.

23. Levine C. Military medical research: are there ethical exceptions? *IRB: A Review of Human Subjects Research*. 1989;11(4):5–7.

24. Presidential Advisory Committee on Gulf War Veterans' Illnesses. *Final Report*. Washington, DC: US Government Printing Office; 1996.

25. *Oversight of NIH and FDA: Bioethics and the Adequacy of Informed Consent, 1977: Hearing Before the Human Resources Subcommittee of the House Committee on Government Reform and Oversight*, 105th Cong, 1st Sess (1997).

26. Jonas H. Philosophical reflections on experimenting with human subjects. In: Freund PA, ed. *Experimentation with Human Subjects*. New York, NY: George Braziller; 1970:1–32.

27. Christakis N. Do medical student research subjects need special protection? *IRB: A Review of Human Subjects Research*.1985;7(3):1–4.

28. Kopelman L. Cynicism among medical students. *JAMA*. 1993;250(15):2006–2010.

29. American Psychological Association. Ethical principles of psychologists and code of conduct. http://www.apa.org/ethics/code/principles.pdf. Effective June 1, 2003. Amended June 1, 2010. Accessed December 4, 2017.

30. McNeil D Jr. U.S. apologizes for syphilis tests in Guatemala. *New York Times*. October 1, 2010:B4.

31. Presidential Commission for the Study of Bioethical Issues. *"Ethically Impossible": STD Research in Guatemala from 1946 to 1948*. Washington, DC: US Government Printing Office; 2011. https://law.stanford.edu/wp-content/uploads/2011/09/EthicallyImpossible_PCSBI_110913.pdf//bioethics.gov/sites/default/files/Ethically-Impossible_PCSBI.pdf. Accessed December 4, 2017.

32. Moreno JD. *Mind Wars: Brain Science and the Military in the 21st Century*. New York, NY: Bellevue Literary Press; 2006.

33. Federal policy for the protection of human subjects; final rule. *Federal Register*. 2017;82(12):7149-7246. Available at https://www.gpo.gov/fdsys/pkg/FR-2017-01-19/html/2017-01058.htm. Accessed December 5, 2017.

10 JUSTICE AND GLOBAL RESEARCH

Ruth Macklin

This chapter addresses several interrelated concerns regarding justice in global health research involving human beings. The standard conception of distributive justice requires that the benefits and burdens of research be allocated fairly. The concept of justice always relates to fairness in some way, but there are competing conceptions of how resources should be allocated fairly. Moreover, justice is not limited to the question of fair distribution. Other conceptions of justice address fair procedures[1] and fair compensation. In addition to examining the familiar notion of distributive justice as it applies to global health research, the chapter explores several different conceptions of justice that are also potentially relevant.

Ethical concerns about the conduct of global health research arise primarily because of the economic gap between industrialized countries (the major sponsors of research along with the pharmaceutical industry) and resource-poor countries in which much biomedical research is carried out. Although still commonly used, the terms "developing" and "developed" have become less relevant today than in the past because of the rapid economic development of countries such as Brazil, India, and China, while extremely low-resource countries in sub-Saharan Africa have not seen comparable development. The currently preferred term in the context of global health is "low and middle-income countries" (LMIC). With occasional references to "developing" and "developed" countries (mostly from existing literature), this chapter uses the term "LMIC," along with "low-resource" and "resource-poor," to refer to the poorest countries, and "wealthy" or "industrialized" to refer to richer countries. It should be noted, however, that all of these terms focus on economic development, which may not reflect other important indicators such as the quality of the health system and infrastructure, the level of scientific research conducted by local investigators, and the health literacy of the population.

The chapter explores various views on the acceptability of "double standards"[2] in research. One formulation of a single standard in global health research is the following:

> To meet the requirements of distributive justice in global research, two conditions must be fulfilled:
> - The design and determination of acceptable risk/benefit ratios must be evaluated with the same standards as when such research is carried out in the sponsoring country.
> - Beneficiaries of the research outcomes must include people in the countries where the research is conducted, as well as in the industrialized country that sponsors the research. (p. 78)[3]

These conditions make it clear that it is not only the benefits and burdens accruing to the research participants that count in determining equity, but also the prospect of benefits to the community or the country where the research is carried out.

The discussion of justice in global research is complicated by the existence of different types of benefits, as well as a difference between risk-benefit profiles in different circumstances. Participants in a clinical trial may receive an experimental drug that turns out to benefit them, although that cannot be known in advance. In a prevention study, such as a clinical trial of a vaccine to prevent infection with HIV, participants who become infected during the trial (typically as a result of their risky behavior, not the vaccine itself) may be provided with a proven effective treatment for HIV, which will clearly benefit them; but the benefit will not be from the research interventions themselves. Still another type of benefit is known as "ancillary care": treatment for other medical conditions that may exist alongside whatever is being studied in the research. Examples include treatment for sexually transmitted infections detected during HIV related research and provision of contraception for those enrolled in clinical trials. Finally, post-trial benefits to the country or community could include sponsor provision of successful products of research or other things the community might value.

Justice Over Time

Concerns about justice in research have a long history, going back to the landmark *Belmont Report* in 1979. In explicating what is meant by justice in research that report said, "research should not unduly involve persons from groups unlikely to be among the beneficiaries of subsequent applications of the research" (p. 23194).[4] Although the *Belmont Report* was drafted in the context of research conducted in the United States, the principles articulated in that historic document have come to be known throughout the world. Beginning in about 1990, there has been a dramatic increase in the amount of industry-sponsored research in LMIC, giving rise to questions about justice on a global scale. The reasons for this increase are partly economic, since it is generally cheaper to conduct research in places where labor costs are lower. A second reason is that a larger number of people in poor countries are "drug naïve," that is, they have not been exposed to drugs that are widely used in wealthier countries and this is an advantage in testing experimental medications. Furthermore, in the early years of the increase it was easier to get research protocols approved in countries that did not have well-established research ethics committees. That situation has since improved with the introduction of training programs and capacity building for ethics in research that have occurred over the past ten to fifteen years. The Fogarty International Center of the US National Institutes of Health (NIH) has sponsored training programs in research ethics in an initiative begun in 2000. Directors of these programs have come from both the United States and resource-poor countries. Another set of capacity-building programs in research ethics has been sponsored by the Department of Bioethics at the NIH Clinical Center. In addition, several departments at the World Health Organization (WHO) have conducted similar programs. However, it remains true that neither the majority of the population nor the governments in resource-poor countries can afford the cost of all successful products of research that become available in industrialized countries.

Early concerns about justice in global health research focused mostly on risks, specifically, the lack of mechanisms in place in low-resource countries to protect the rights and welfare of the research participants. A major concern was the risk of exploitation, understood here as follows: "Exploitation occurs when wealthy or powerful individuals or agencies take advantage of the poverty, powerlessness, or dependency of others by using the latter to serve their own ends (those of the wealthy or powerful) without adequate compensating benefits for the less powerful or disadvantaged individuals or groups" (p. 101–102).[5] Examples could include inadequate methods for obtaining informed consent, and using poorly trained research ethics committees that would readily approve research proposals. Although concerns about risks to subjects have not entirely disappeared, more recent ethical concerns have focused on the provision of benefits to subjects and to the community, largely as a result of what has transpired in the AIDS epidemic, at the beginning of which no treatment existed outside the research context. A shift then occurred from the perception of research as a risky endeavor to one that can yield significant benefits to research subjects and the wider community when research results in successful products or other interventions. Both of these concerns—inadequate protection of risks to research subjects and the absence of any benefits—constitute a violation of distributive justice that calls for an equitable distribution of research burdens and benefits.[4] Moreover, a principle of equity requires that no single group—gender, racial, ethnic, geographic, or socioeconomic—receives disproportionate benefits or bears disproportionate burdens.[5]

Risk-Benefit Ratios

As noted above, different risk-benefit profiles may exist in different countries or regions, thereby complicating judgments about what justice requires. The formal principle of justice—"treat like cases alike"—can be interpreted to mean that if a study design is the same in two different countries, then if it is unethical in one place, it is unethical in the other. The problem in applying this formal principle is that it is sometimes difficult to determine whether the situations are relevantly similar or relevantly different.

Guidelines and recommendations often refer to ethical standards, a notion that seems clear on its face but requires explication. An influential ethics guidance document issued by the Council for International Organizations of Medical Sciences (CIOMS) makes the following point: "[In some settings] resources are so limited that the population may be vulnerable to exploitation by sponsors and investigators from wealthier countries and communities. The ethical standards applied should be no less stringent than they would be for research carried out in high-resource settings" (Commentary, Guideline 2).[6] Here, as elsewhere, the concept of ethical standards remains unanalyzed. This vagueness gives rise to two problems. The first is failure to distinguish between principled ethical standards, on the one hand, and ethically necessary procedural mechanisms, on the other. The second problem is uncertainty whether ethical standards for research should be universally applicable or whether they may be relative to cultural norms, and economic or other differences among countries. The answer to both questions depends on what counts as an ethical standard. As one article queries: "Does what is provided to a control group in a randomized, controlled trial—often referred to as standard of care—count as a standard? Does the level of treatment provided to research participants in the course of a trial constitute an ethical standard? Are the requirements for the manner in which informed consent is obtained and documented ethical standards? Or are they procedures, important yet properly distinguishable from principled ethical standards?" (p. 12).[7]

Whatever might be meant by "ethical standards," worries about justice in global health research revolve around the question of double standards—one for wealthier countries and another for resource-poor countries.[2] One candidate for a universal standard in research ethics might be the following: *If it is unethical to carry out a particular research project in an industrialized country, it would be unethical to do that same research in a resource-poor country.* Although appealing, this formulation is flawed because it fails to recognize that particular circumstances can be so different that some research that could not be conducted in an industrialized country could still be ethically acceptable in a developing country. The three examples (placebo controls, rotavirus vaccines, and RU-486) that follow demonstrate the difficulty that can arise in determining whether the circumstances in industrialized countries and LMIC are relevantly similar or different, and thus whether research in the low-income setting is just or unjust.

The Controversy over Placebos

A landmark episode that launched debate in the medical and bioethics literature was a clinical trial carried out in developing countries in the 1990s. The NIH and US Centers for Disease Control and Prevention (CDC) sponsored trials to see whether a short-course regimen of azidothymidine (AZT), a medication already shown to be effective in industrialized countries, would reduce transmission of HIV from infected pregnant women to their offspring. The control group in the developing countries received a placebo, which could not have been used in the industrialized countries where an effective intervention existed and was available to pregnant HIV–infected women. Defenders of the trials argued that by receiving a placebo the women in the developing country trials received the "standard of care" (that is, no effective preventive method since none was generally available to these women), so placebo controls were ethically acceptable. Critics contended that withholding an effective treatment not only was unethical, as it failed to minimize the risk of HIV transmission from mother to child, but the trial design also violated a provision in the most prominent international ethical guidance, the Declaration of Helsinki (DoH).[8] This episode prompted a strong response by researchers, sponsors, and bioethicists, and led to a protracted effort to revise the DoH. Defenders of the placebo-controlled trials did not want to be seen as violating a major international guideline for research, so they urged a revision of the DoH that would weaken the provision requiring that a proven treatment always be given to the control group.

The opposing sides in this dispute could both claim that justice was on their side. Critics began with the premise that the same study could not ethically be carried out in developed countries and concluded that, therefore, it would be unethical to conduct it in developing countries. The sponsoring agencies and other supporters of the study began with the premise that risk-benefit ratios are radically different in the resource-poor countries where the research was conducted and in the United States, the sponsoring country. In the United States, almost all pregnant women potentially had access to the effective regimen but in the low-resource countries, very few or none did. In the resource-poor countries, subjects were not being placed at greater risk than if they were not in the study at all, and many more people could potentially benefit much sooner from the results of a shorter, placebo-controlled trial. Therefore, it could be argued, the principle "treat like cases alike" was not violated since the two situations were not similar, but differed in relevant respects. Furthermore, since the short-course regimen of AZT was designed specifically for resource-poor countries, the potential benefits would accrue specifically to that population, so an important feature of equity would be fulfilled: the same population undergoing the risks would be the recipient of benefits of the research. In reply, critics maintained that the control group could have been provided with the proven preventive method, so risks of transmitting HIV from mother to child would be drastically reduced. This viewpoint rests on a fundamental ethical obligation in research to minimize risks to the subjects.

The debate prompted by this episode has not disappeared. Controversy continues over whether justice requires a single, worldwide standard in the conduct of research, or whether "double standards," based on economic, social, or cultural differences, are ethically permissible. According to the "single standard" position, one global standard must prevail for research to be considered just. The opposing position maintains that as long as what is provided to research subjects conforms to what is available to the general population in a country or region, such studies meet an acceptable standard of justice.

Studying a Rotavirus Vaccine

A telling example of a difference in the risk-benefit ratio is that of a rotavirus vaccine that was licensed in the United States based on clinical trials conducted in the United States and Finland. Rotavirus causes serious diarrheal disease and claims the lives of a huge number of children in developing countries—approximately 600,000 to 800,000 annually. After the vaccine was licensed in the United States, it was discovered to cause intussusception, a serious disorder in which intestinal obstruction occurs and can be fatal. If treated promptly, the condition can be cured with no lasting effects. After this serious side effect was discovered, the CDC recommended postponing the vaccination of children in the United States and the manufacturer voluntarily withdrew the vaccine from the market in the United States. This action prompted the question whether the vaccine should be tested in developing countries. If it caused this serious condition in children, could it be ethically acceptable to conduct clinical trials in developing countries to determine its safety and efficacy in those settings? An uncritical acceptance of the position that the product was unsafe for children in the United States so it would be unethical to conduct trials in developing countries fails to take into account differences in the risk-benefit profiles. In the United States, the number of children who died annually from rotavirus diarrhea was only about twenty, while the virus caused hundreds of thousands of deaths of children in low-income countries. According to one account: "Assuming a worst case scenario of a 25% fatality rate from intussusception in developing countries, widespread use of tetravalent rhesus rotavirus vaccine could cause 2000–3000 deaths a year" (p. 525).[9] These tragic deaths stand in stark contrast to the hundreds of thousands of deaths from the virus in low-resource countries. It is evident that a simple formula such as "If it is unethical in the United States it would be unethical in a developing country" is insufficiently nuanced to serve as a benchmark for determining ethical standards.

Clinical Trials of RU-486 in Bangladesh

RU-486, an agent used for early pregnancy termination, was initially tested in Europe in research carried out by the WHO. A great need exists for affordable and safe abortion in LMIC, but abortion remains illegal in the majority of such countries. Although abortion has been illegal in Bangladesh, the procedure known as "menstrual regulation" remained legal. As long as a woman was not tested for pregnancy, products that could "bring on menses" were used without question or legal interference. Given that situation in Bangladesh, RU-486, a proven abortifacient, was proposed for trials there. However, two prominent women's health advocates objected to the initiation of clinical trials of RU-486 in Bangladesh. They argued that the compound had been demonstrated to be an effective method of choice for a substantial number of women in France, a country with a strong health infrastructure. In Bangladesh, a country with weak health and family planning infrastructures, women would be likely to undergo greater risks both during clinical trials and after introduction of this method than they faced in the use of the menstrual regulation techniques then currently employed. These advocates recommended conducting trials in several industrialized countries and possibly in selected low-resource countries where strong health infrastructures exist: "Before women in Southern countries with weak health services are exposed to the risks of RU-486/PG [prostaglandin, part of the pregnancy termination protocol], it is our strong view that, for health as well as political reasons, RU-486/PG must be further researched in several Northern countries especially the US. . . ."[10]

On the other side of this debate are those who argued that questioning the wisdom of conducting studies of RU-486 in particular settings inappropriately denies women a beneficial option. In this debate, both sides appealed to considerations of justice. Those who favored instituting the trials argued that to deny Bangladeshi women the benefits of RU-486 would be unjust. Those opposed contended that to subject Bangladeshi women to risks greater than they faced in their present situation would be unjust. Interestingly, extensive trials of an RU-486 analog, sponsored by the WHO, were conducted in China, then considered a low-resource country. But unlike Bangladesh, China had a well-developed health infrastructure so the objections to conducting the trials in Bangladesh would not apply to China.

These differences in risk-benefit assessments from one country to the next demonstrate the difficulty in trying to apply the rule, "If it is unethical to carry out a particular research project in an industrialized country, it would be unethical to do that same research in a resource-poor country." The relevant principle of justice is "treat like cases alike, in relevant respects." China and Bangladesh were alike in that they both were developing countries, yet they were unlike in respect to the risk-benefit profile of clinical trials. China's better health infrastructure yielded a different risk-benefit ratio from Bangladesh's poor systems of medical research and service delivery. In respects relevant to assessing the risks and benefits of the research, even years ago China was more like France and the UK than it was like Bangladesh.

Post-trial Benefits to Participants and the Community

What does justice require when industrialized countries or industry sponsor and conduct research in resource-poor countries? Diverse interpretations of justice and related concepts are one source of controversy regarding what—if anything—industrialized country sponsors owe to research subjects, to the community, or to the country as a whole when research yields successful products or contributions to knowledge. More specifically, do sponsors of research conducted in resource-poor countries have an obligation to provide the successful products of research when clinical trials are concluded? When research is carried out in industrialized countries, a reasonable expectation exists that both the research subjects and the general population will have access to successful interventions, either through the mechanism of private insurance or through medical care provided by the government. Key provisions in leading international ethical guidelines address post-trial benefits to the community or country where the research is carried out; an alternative view is a critique known as "the fair benefits framework."[11] These positions are discussed further below.

International Ethical Guidelines for Research

What do the leading international ethical guidelines say about what is owed to research subjects and to others at the conclusion of a trial? All of the relevant ethics guidance documents express the general idea that research should be responsive to the health needs of the population where the research is conducted and should potentially benefit that population in some way. But beyond this basic agreement, viewpoints diverge in several ways.

Consider first the DoH. Issued by the World Medical Association (WMA), the DoH has been adopted as an ethics reference document for research with human subjects by many countries. First issued in a rather skeletal form in 1964 and after having undergone mostly minor changes beginning in 1975, the DoH underwent a major revision in 2000 primarily in response to the controversy over the placebo-controlled HIV studies in pregnant women described earlier in this chapter. Earlier versions did not include any statements expressing a general requirement for making successful products available to research subjects or to others. The 2000 revision, however, addressed the point in two separate paragraphs, 19 and 30. Paragraph 19 said, "Medical research is only justified if there is a reasonable likelihood that the populations in which the research is carried out stand to benefit from the results of the research."[12] The brevity of the statement and the absence of any commentary or explication leave crucial questions wide open. For example, what are the criteria by which "likelihood of benefit" is to be determined? And what degree of likelihood is necessary? The 2000 revision of the DoH also addressed the question of benefits to the subject population in a strongly worded requirement in paragraph 30: "At the conclusion of the study, every patient entered into the study should be assured of access to the best proven prophylactic, diagnostic and therapeutic methods identified by the study."[12]

Beginning with the 2000 revision, the DoH has been subjected to more scrutiny than it had experienced in the previous decades of its existence. The WMA embarked on another revision culminating in 2008. One can only speculate whether powerful forces exerted pressure on the WMA to change some key provisions that were viewed as unfriendly to industry and major governmental sponsors of global health research. A change in wording in the paragraph describing post-trial benefits may at first appear minor. The 2008 version says at paragraph 33: "At the conclusion of the study, patients entered into the study are entitled to be informed about the outcome of the study and to share any benefits that result from it, for example, access to interventions identified as beneficial in the study or to other appropriate care or benefits."[13] Are the ethical implications of this version stronger or weaker than those of the earlier version? The 2000 version does not mention informing participants about the outcome of the study, so that supports an argument that the later version is stronger. In addition, the earlier version says that participants should be "assured of access" to methods identified by the study. But "assuring" people that they will have access is not at all the same as "ensuring access" to such methods. Nevertheless, it is possible to read the earlier version as promising more to participants than the 2008 version. The latter cites access to interventions only as "an example" of benefits resulting from the study. There may be "other appropriate care or benefits," according to the new DoH. But what might they be? And how to determine what is *appropriate* care or benefits? Interpretation of these paragraphs of the DoH are left to whatever bodies, be they research ethics committees or sponsors, seek to implement the provisions of the DoH. That document was revised yet again in 2013, and the provision for post-trial benefits to study participants was restored to its earlier strong position in paragraph 34: "In advance of a clinical trial, sponsors, researchers and host country governments should make provisions for post-trial access for all participants who still need an intervention identified as beneficial in the trial. This information must also be disclosed to participants during the informed consent process."[8] An important addition in this revision is the inclusion of responsibilities of the host country government, typically the Ministry of Health in LMIC. This wording implies that even resource-poor countries should be prepared to share in making the benefits of research available to the participants in clinical trials.

Unlike the DoH, which contains rather brief statements of its principles, the CIOMS international ethical guidelines[6] include a rather detailed commentary under each guideline. CIOMS underwent revision from its 1993 version at about the same time as the DoH was being revised in response to the placebo debate. The 2002 revised CIOMS document contains both a general statement of responsiveness to the health needs of the population, and also the explicit requirement that successful products be made "reasonably available" to the population. Both points are included in Guideline 10:

> Before undertaking research in a population or community with limited resources, the sponsor and the researcher must make every effort to ensure that:
> - the research is responsive to the health needs and the priorities of the population or community in which it is to be carried out; and
> - any product developed will be made reasonably available to that population or community.[6]

Aside from the substantive content of this CIOMS guideline, the use of the active rather than the passive voice renders it superior to the corresponding paragraph in earlier versions of the DoH because CIOMS identifies the responsible agents: the sponsor and the researcher. Even when not mentioned explicitly, the assumption that the researcher and sponsor are responsible for making post-trial benefits available underlies much of the discussion on this point. However, that assumption has been criticized by Pratt and Loff,[14] who argue that it places responsibility on the wrong actors. These authors contend that the proper agents are governments, not sponsors of research or the investigators conducting the research. While this is a significant criticism of CIOMS and other documents that call for sponsors and researchers to bear the burden of justice in research by ensuring that developing countries receive the benefits of successful research, Pratt and Loff's objection is nowhere near as critical as that of proponents of the "fair benefits" framework (see a discussion of this position in the next section).

Two other international ethics guidance documents discuss post-trial access to successful products of research as matters of justice. These documents address only one specific type of research: HIV biomedical prevention research. Despite their focus on only one type of research for a particular disease, these guidance documents are instructive for their respective approaches. The first, guidance issued by UNAIDS and the WHO,[15] does not explicitly refer to justice. Yet it contains the strongest statement of any regarding post-trial access. Guidance Point 19, Availability of Outcomes, says: "During the initial stages of development of a biomedical HIV prevention trial, trial sponsors and countries should agree on responsibilities and plans to make available as soon as possible any biomedical HIV preventive intervention demonstrated to be safe and effective . . . to all participants in the trials in which it was tested, as well as to other populations at higher risk of HIV exposure in the country."[15]

This requirement is stronger than those in either CIOMS or the DoH and it mentions both trial participants and the larger community.

The other ethics guidance for research on HIV prevention is issued by the HIV Prevention Trials Network (HPTN, an international collaborative clinical trials network).[16] Its 2009 revision of its guidelines refers explicitly to social justice, explaining that for the purpose of this ethical guidance, the concept "expresses the ethical concerns related to treating people equally, avoiding exploitation, and trying to reduce health disparities" (p. 14).[16] Guidance Point 15 addresses post-trial access: "HPTN research seeking to establish the efficacy of an intervention must have a preliminary plan regarding the provision of successful interventions to research participants and communities."[16] The HPTN guidance distinguishes between "ethical obligations" and what it calls "ethical aspirations." The distinction is explained as follows. "If a course of action is described as an ethical obligation (expressed in terms such as 'should,' 'must' or 'will'), then normally the action should be done, and while exceptions to that course of action are permissible, these exceptions require a strong ethical justification. . . . In contrast, a course of action expressed in terms of an *ethical aspiration* (expressed in terms such as 'making good faith efforts') implies that following the course of action is admirable or commendable—a matter of pursuing important ethical ideals—but is not required" (p. 12).[16] In Guidance Point 15, "making *plans* regarding the provision of successful interventions to participants" is treated as an ethical obligation, whereas "provision of successful interventions to participants, communities and at-risk populations" is considered an ethical aspiration (p. 59).[16] This distinction is appealing to critics of the CIOMS and UNAIDS/WHO ethical guidance, both of which contain strong statements about ensuring post-trial access to successful products of research.

The Fair Benefits Framework

Guideline 10 of the CIOMS international guidelines was targeted for criticism by participants at a 2001 conference on ethical aspects of research in developing countries.[11,17] The critique, known as the "fair benefits framework" (the "Framework") begins with the claim that making successful products of research available to the community or country is not necessary for benefits to be equitable. The Framework claims that this is chiefly because benefits other than the successful products of research may be valued equally, if not more, by the community where research is conducted. While that may well be the case, it ignores the main purpose of conducting research in LMIC: to obtain knowledge that can benefit the health of that population. The critique contains a series of separate points leading to the conclusion that benefits other than that of the successful products of research are fair and may be ethically superior to provision of the product itself.[18] One point is the contention that the specification of benefits in the CIOMS guideline is too narrow. The critique says that other potential benefits could include training persons who provide health services or construction of clinics, hospitals, or other physical infrastructure. This point is well taken, but only if successful products were the only possible or allowable benefit. A requirement to make the products of research available does not preclude the possibility of also providing other benefits to the community.

Another of the Framework's objections to the CIOMS guideline is the charge of paternalism. The critique claims that it is paternalistic for the sponsor or ethical guidelines to specify what ought to be the benefits of research. It implies that officials or the population in the country cannot make their own autonomous decisions. The charge of paternalism is rather odd, as it is the nature of ethical recommendations that they are paternalistic. Many requirements in ethical guidelines dictate what ought to be done; such guidelines often name the responsible agents for ensuring the ethical conduct of research and may include researchers, sponsors, research ethics committees, and governmental oversight agencies. As for the population in the community or country making its "own autonomous decision," this suggestion is fraught with practical problems. For one thing, it would be necessary to establish a mechanism by which the population could choose the benefits of research. Beyond that, it is unrealistic to suppose that the population in low-resource countries or communities could negotiate its preferred set of benefits with a powerful pharmaceutical company sponsoring the research. Although community consultation or engagement is desirable and even considered mandatory in some ethics guidance for research, the disparity in power between the population in a resource-poor setting and the other main actors (sponsors of research and governmental officials) is a formidable obstacle to truly democratic decision-making.

The fair benefits critique ignores the public health purpose of conducting biomedical research: to prevent, cure, or ameliorate diseases in human beings. If research does, in fact, yield successful products, and these are not made available to the population in a resource-poor country but are accessible to people in wealthier countries, it is not only unjust, but also prompts the question of what is the ethical justification for conducting the research in the developing country in the first place. As one article notes, ". . . if the results of a clinical trial are not made reasonably available in a timely manner to study participants and other inhabitants of a host country, the researchers might be justly accused of exploiting poor, undereducated subjects for the benefit of more affluent populations of the sponsoring countries" (p. 29).[19]

Procedural Justice: The Role of Ethical Review Committees

One mechanism for seeking to ensure justice in the application of ethical standards to international collaborative research is that of review by committees in both the sponsoring country and the host country. The US governmental regulations for ethics in research are almost entirely procedural, and unlike the DoH and the CIOMS international guidelines, the US regulations do not include any provisions related to research design (the use of placebo controls) or to post-trial benefits. Research ethics committees can introduce their own procedural requirements beyond what the US federal regulations require. This emphasis on procedures can lead to some peculiar results, as illustrated in the following example.

An example in which an institutional review board (IRB) in the United States sought to impose its own requirements on a research study from another country illustrates the importance of understanding cross-cultural differences while at the same time maintaining high ethical standards. The researcher, a social scientist from Latin America, was collaborating on a project with a social scientist from the United States and the protocol was reviewed at the North American researcher's institution. The research was a study of forms of coercion in sexual relations among adolescents, ranging from efforts by male adolescents to persuade their girlfriends to have sex to cases of forcible rape. In an exhibition of "political correctness" the IRB insisted that the Latin American investigator define as "coercive" any situation in which a female adolescent at first says "no" to sex but eventually agrees. The investigator sought to explain the cultural context, in which sexual relations among adolescents are socially condemned in her country by adults, who deny the prevalence of adolescent sexuality. The society is undergoing changes. A female adolescent who is entirely willing to have sex with her boyfriend—and there are many—must nevertheless adhere to the mores that dictate she must first refuse, even adamantly, lest she appear to be promiscuous. The IRB refused to acknowledge the reality of this cultural difference, maintaining its insistence on the American criterion for sexual harassment: "No means no." This was an attempt by the IRB to alter the methodology of the research by assuming the universality of a cultural norm applicable to the United States but not to Latin America.[20]

In its review of the same study, the IRB sought to impose on the investigator a requirement to report to the police and to parents cases in which female adolescents told the researcher they had been raped. The Latin American researcher argued vehemently against this proposed requirement on several grounds: (1) reporting to parents or the police would violate the confidentiality the researcher promised the subjects; (2) rape victims in her country are further victimized by the police, who are not appropriately trained and who maintain that women must have been acting in a way to provoke the rape; (3) parents may also blame the victim and, in addition, because they are likely to feel shame when confronted by a stranger (the researcher) about such an intimate matter, they may take further punitive action against the young woman; and (4) the episodes reported to the researcher by subjects would have occurred sufficiently long ago that it would be impossible to do physical examinations or take additional steps that might lead to apprehension and conviction of the rapist. The researcher in this case complained about the inappropriateness of IRB review in the United States of a study she sought to conduct in her own country in Latin America. However, the review itself is not inappropriate since the aim is to ensure that internationally agreed-upon ethical standards are adhered to in global health research. What was inappropriate was the IRB's flawed insistence on identical procedures to those that would be used in such cases in the United States without being sensitive to the local context in which the proposed research was to take place.

This example illustrates the difference between substantive ethical standards of justice and ethical procedures in global health research. The application of different ethical standards to different countries or regions can result in an injustice, as the existence of double standards invariably implies higher and lower standards, and not merely different standards. In contrast, variation in procedural mechanisms in research need not imply an injustice in ethical standards. Procedures such as those illustrated in the above example may vary according to customs, locally available infrastructure, or other circumstances without violating principles of justice that require equal respect for human beings participating in global research.

Looking Ahead

Several procedural steps can aid in the attempt to secure justice in global health research. The first is genuine collaboration between researchers in industrialized countries or in international agencies, such as the WHO, that sponsor or carry out clinical research. Genuine collaboration requires research training and joint efforts, instead of allowing North American or European scientists direct access to populations in developing countries, as occurred in the past. Current guidelines for global health research call for including mechanisms to assist developing countries in building capacity for research. Researchers from developing countries are seeking greater recognition of their collaborative roles, especially in coauthorship of publications resulting from their research.

A second step is to incorporate more fully the requirement of community involvement in the research process, which is stated in several ethics guidance documents. This includes community consultation or consensus before and during the conduct of the research, and also a determination that the community or region is likely to benefit in some way from the research outcomes. A requirement of community consultation has evolved as a feature of AIDS research both in the United States and globally, but is not yet fully realized (see Chapter 8).

The attainment of justice in any sphere requires both the application of substantive principles of justice and the establishment of procedural mechanisms such as those described briefly here. As illustrated in this chapter, justice in global health research cannot be analyzed separately from the more familiar concerns of assessing the risks and benefits of research and evaluating relevant similarities and differences among wealthier and poorer countries. Although justice has not occupied center stage in earlier discussions of global health research ethics in the past, it is a critical aspect in today's global context.

International guidelines applicable to countries throughout the world seek to achieve justice by ensuring the universal applicability of ethical requirements of research involving human subjects. However, as demonstrated in this chapter, principles of justice may be open to different and conflicting interpretations, and disagreement can arise over their correct application. There is no single principle of justice, but *fairness* remains the underlying value.

As theories of social justice and justice in health have become more numerous in recent years,[21,22,23] bioethicists, political theorists, human rights lawyers, and philosophers have articulated different accounts of what is owed to resource-poor countries. An examination of those theories is beyond the scope of this chapter. But it is clear that attention to global justice is here to stay. Since transnational research is now a global enterprise, rectifying injustices in global research is a moral imperative.

Notes

1. Daniels N. Accountability for reasonableness: establishing a fair process for priority setting is easier than agreeing on principles. *BMJ*. 2000;321(7272):1300–1301.
2. Macklin R. *Double Standards in Biomedical Research in Developing Countries*. Cambridge, England: Cambridge University Press; 2004.

3. Mastroianni A, Faden R, Federman D, eds. *Women and Health Research: Ethical and Legal Issues of Including Women in Clinical Studies*. Vol. 1. Washington, DC: National Academy Press; 1994.

4. National Commission for the Protection of Human Subjects of Biomedical and Behavioral Research. The Belmont Report: Ethical principles and guidelines for the protection of human subjects of research. *Federal Register*. 1979;44(76):23192–23197.

5. Macklin R. *Double Standards in Medical Research in Developing Countries*. Cambridge, England: Cambridge University Press; 2004.

6. Council for International Organizations of Medical Sciences (CIOMS); World Health Organization. International Ethical Guidelines for Health-Related Research Involving Humans. Geneva, Switzerland: CIOMS; 2016. https://cioms. ch/wp-content/uploads/2017/01/WEB-CIOMS-EthicalGuidelines.pdf. Accessed December 4, 2017.

7. Macklin R. Appropriate ethical standards. In: Emanuel EJ, Grady CC, Crouch RA, Lie RK, Miller FG, Wendler, DD, eds. *The Oxford Textbook of Clinical Research Ethics*. New York, NY: Oxford University Press; 2008:711–718.

8. World Medical Association. Declaration of Helsinki: ethical principles for medical research involving human subjects. https://www.wma.net/policies-post/ wma-declaration-of-helsinki-ethical-principles-for-medical-research-involving-human-subjects/ . Updated October 2013. Accessed November 30, 2017.

9. Weijer C. The future of research into rotavirus vaccine. *BMJ*. 2000;321(7260):525.

10. Kabir SM, Germain A. Is RU-486/PG in its current form likely to be appropriate for women in Bangladesh? In: Kamal GM, ed. *Proceedings of the International Symposium on Antiprogestins*. Dhaka, Bangladesh: Bangladesh Association for Prevention of Septic Abortion; 1992:48–57.

11. Participants in the 2001 Conference on Ethical Aspects of Research in Developing Countries. Fair benefits for research in developing countries [Ethics]. *Science*. 2002;298(5601):2133–2134.

12. World Medical Association. Declaration of Helsinki: ethical principles for medical research involving human subjects. Version 2000. http://www.who.int/bulletin/archives/79(4)373.pdf. Accessed November 30, 2017.

13. World Medical Association. Declaration of Helsinki: ethical principles for medical research involving human subjects. Version 2008. https://www.wma.net/ what-we-do/medical-ethics/declaration-of-helsinki/doh-oct2008/. Accessed November 30, 2017.

14. Pratt B, Loff B. Justice in international clinical research. *Developing World Bioethics*. 2011;11(2):75–81.

15. Joint United Nations Programme on HIV/AIDS (UNAIDS); World Health Organization (WHO). *Ethical Considerations in Biomedical HIV Prevention Trials* (UNAIDS/WHO guidance document). Geneva, Switzerland: UNAIDS; 2012. http:// files.unaids.org/en/media/unaids/contentassets/documents/unaidspublication/ 2012/jc1399_ethical_considerations_en.pdf. Accessed November 30, 2017.

16. Rennie SJ, Sugarman J. HPTN Ethics Working Group. Ethics guidance for research. https://www.hptn.org/about/ethics. Revised 2009. Accessed November 30, 2017.

17. Participants in the 2001 Conference on Ethical Aspects of Research in Developing Countries. Moral standards for research in developing countries: from "reasonable availability" to "fair benefits." *Hastings Center Report.* 2004;34(3):17–27.

18. Macklin R. Intertwining biomedical research and public health in HIV preventive microbicide research. *Public Health Ethics.* 2010;3(3):199–209.

19. Crouch RA, Arras JD. AZT trials and tribulations. *Hastings Center Report.* 1998;28(6):26–34.

20. This episode was told to me by a colleague who requested anonymity.

21. Daniels N. *Just Health: Meeting Health Needs Fairly.* Cambridge, England: Cambridge University Press; 2008.

22. Ruger JP. *Health and Social Justice.* New York, NY: Oxford University Press; 2010.

23. Powers M, Faden R. *Social Justice.* New York, NY: Oxford University Press; 2006.

11 THEORIZING JUSTICE IN HEALTH RESEARCH

Yashar Saghai

Although several theories of justice have been developed exclusively for or have a major focus on health care, public health, and health policy,[1-5] they surprisingly do not include an explicit focus on health research. Instead, theoretical considerations of justice have informed debates on health research ethics primarily through discussions of principles of distributive justice and, more recently, principles of nonoppression and nondomination. These principles and related concepts (such as disadvantage, exploitation, vulnerability, and solidarity) have been applied to health research issues that have an identifiable justice dimension.

In this chapter, I pursue two goals. The first is to critically examine the meanings and roles of various *principles* of justice in research ethics contexts that have been discussed in this volume and highlight some of the most promising lines of inquiry that are likely to persist and deepen over the coming years. The second is to make the case for a complementary, but significantly different, approach: to gauge the extent to which current *theories* (rather than principles) of justice might be systematically mobilized, expanded, and specified to build relevant and sophisticated approaches to justice in health research, domestically and globally. Such a theoretical move might be advantageous for articulating a coherent approach to the range of issues that come under the "health research" heading, broadly construed, including research in basic biomedical sciences, clinical settings, public health, health policy, social determinants of health, health systems, and health-focused social and behavioral sciences.

Debates on Principles of Justice in Health Research

In this section I discuss the main principles of justice that have played, and continue to play, a major role in research ethics debates, namely, principles of distributive justice and principles of nonoppression and nondomination. Though principles of distributive justice were at first used to protect subjects from the potential harm of research, those principles were next mobilized to increase access to the benefits of research. Nonoppression and nondomination are more recent "umbrella" principles of research ethics that are attentive to pervasive structures of domination and related power imbalances, which are irreducible to distributive concerns.

The Belmont Report *and Principles of Distributive Justice in Subject Selection*

Although issues of justice in health research were brought to the forefront of public debate in the United States before the publication in 1979 of the *Belmont Report* by the US National Commission for the Protection of Human Subjects of Biomedical and Behavioral Research, it is arguably *Belmont* that framed the debate in formal justice language.[6-8] Against a historical background of grave injustices toward members of vulnerable populations, the *Belmont Report* claims that subject selection should be guided by principles of distributive justice, that is, moral norms providing guidance for fair procedures and substantive criteria for the allocation of burdens/risks and benefits/opportunities.

As a starting point, the *Belmont Report* assumes that any departure from egalitarian distributions among parties is in need of justification. Unequal distributions are justified only if they satisfy a formal principle of justice (like cases ought to be treated alike) and a material principle of justice (identifying morally relevant differences between parties). The *Belmont Report* cites several examples of criteria that might plausibly specify material principles of distributive justice in different contexts: age, experience, merit, effort, deprivation, need, and societal contribution.

Importantly, the *Belmont Report* does not endorse any single principle of distributive justice. Rather, its strategy is to rule out criteria for the selection of individuals or groups in health research that, if endorsed, would lead to injustice. These criteria include social undesirability, availability (e.g., prisoners, institutionalized patients), manipulability, and vulnerabilities of various sorts (e.g., those associated with "social, racial, sexual, and cultural biases institutionalized in society").

The *Belmont Report* also claims that social justice requires that entire classes of subjects should not disproportionally bear the burdens of research relative to its benefits, even if individuals within those groups have given valid consent to research. The central concern here is with the potential for exploitation of research subjects who might be taken unfair advantage of, although the term "exploitation" is used only once in this regard when referencing Nazi experiments on unwilling prisoners. Exploitation is sometimes combined with wrongs caused by lack of, or deficiencies in, informed consent. However, the *Belmont Report*'s concern goes clearly beyond consent issues. Its position is in sharp contrast with classical liberal and libertarian conceptions of justice.[9] The defenders of these conceptions[10,11] deny that patterns of distribution of benefits and burdens are morally significant, no matter how unequal they are. They do not concede that the demands of justice go beyond the protection of autonomous choice from fraud or coercion, and see no harm in consensual forms of exploitation.

The *Belmont Report*'s conception of justice and its focus on distributive justice principles leads it to advocate a protective approach to subject selection within the mandate of the National Commission, which was geared toward the protection of the rights and interests of biomedical and behavioral research subjects. The *Belmont* principles were soon translated into basic US federal research regulations.[12] This protective approach has been undeniably serviceable in shielding certain populations from burdens and risks associated with research. However, since the mid-1980s debates on the regulation of research and principles of justice have been reignited, with a move from protection from the potential harm of research to access to the potential benefits of research (see, e.g., Chapter 3).[13] In the following sections I explore some of these debates focusing on the way principles of justice have been deployed to contest or modify the protective approach.

Distributive Justice-Based Arguments for the Right to Participate in Research

One strand of a justice-based critique of the protective approach advocates for the right of research participants to decide what level of burdens/risks and benefits/opportunities is individually acceptable to them. It is tempting to view this trend as a simple revival of the classical liberal or libertarian conception of justice in research because it seems, at first glance, to limit the ethical obligations of researchers and other parties to respect for the autonomous consent of informed adults. This is, however, emphatically not the case. This line of critique of the protective approach is theoretically, and has been historically, compatible with the acknowledgment that the distribution of burdens/ risks and benefits/opportunities among groups matters too.

The point can be made by turning to the rich history of patient advocacy groups that have challenged barriers to access to investigational drugs. This movement started in the 1980s with AIDS advocacy. It was both antipaternalistic and sensitive to social justice. As Steven Epstein has argued, antipaternalistic claims that sponsors, investigators, regulators, and institutional review boards (IRBs) should not substitute their judgments for individuals' own informed evaluation of risks and benefits came hand in hand with the justice concern that research itself is potentially a benefit that should be shared on the basis of need, rather than the ability to pay, like libertarians would posit.[14]

Building on patient advocacy movements, the idea of a right to the benefits of research was later expanded to cover individuals' and communities' right to post-trial benefits (including, according to some, a say on what those benefits should be). This question has become prominent in debates over the exploitation of research participants, especially in international research conducted in low- and middle-income countries (see Chapter 10).[15-17]

In a nutshell, we need to use caution in interpreting the often-described move from protection to participation, which includes but is not limited to debates and regulatory decisions as to which populations should be labeled "vulnerable," and what judgments of vulnerability entail (see Chapter 6). As the protective model was not solely based on concerns for social justice but also on concerns for autonomy, the participative approach is not exclusively based on autonomy. It is often animated by a deep social justice ethos.

Principles of Nonoppression and Nondomination

Despite its importance, the distributive frame misses some important considerations of justice that are not narrowly focused on distributing goods of some kind. This line of argument is extremely influential in thinking about justice issues in health research and comes under different labels, such as principles of nonoppression and nondomination.

In that regard, the work of Iris Marion Young is seminal.[18] It is informed by the justice claims of various social movements (including feminism) and provides conceptual tools for analyzing the limits of the distributive frame. Young argues that by highlighting the burdens and benefits that individuals have to shoulder, distribution-focused theories of justice contribute to obscuring the role of institutional contexts in generating oppression and domination.

The concepts of oppression and domination are central to her thesis. "By domination I mean structural or systemic phenomena which exclude people from participating in determining their actions or the conditions of their actions" (p. 31).[18] In a parallel and influential literature, Philip Pettit construes domination as arbitrary or unchecked control over another's choice.[19] According to Young, oppression is a broader term that overlaps with domination and encompasses exploitation, marginalization, powerlessness, cultural imperialism, and violence.[18] Structural injustices occur when social processes and institutions established by powerful actors serve as background institutional rules and accepted social norms. These rules and norms are imposed on large groups of persons who are not powerful in these same ways. However, powerful actors do not generally have any direct causal responsibility for social injustices of this sort. Their responsibility is indirect: they contribute to create or maintain unjust social structures, and they draw many benefits from the *status quo* and their interactions with other powerful actors under favorable institutional and social design.

Principles of nonoppression and nondomination have changed the lens through which justice issues are framed in health contexts to stress aspects of social relationships that otherwise go unnoticed. However, the future of approaches using these concepts depends on the careful use of several distinctions. First, conflicting conceptions of nonoppression and nondomination need to be explicitly articulated.[19,20] Second, these conceptions should be connected to other moral and political demands and aspirational ideals. Third, explicit and justified statements as to whether, why, and how various actors have specific responsibilities for preventing, resisting, removing, or minimizing structures of oppression and domination in research contexts are necessary. Finally, arguments are needed to vindicate or rebut the claim that the structures of contemporary international health research systematically wrong participants or researchers in low- and middle-income countries. The following examples illustrate this point.

These principles of justice shed new light on the economic model dominant since the 1990s in which powerful pharmaceutical companies increasingly offshore research (international multicenter randomized trials) and outsource trial-related tasks to specialized commercial entities, such as contract research organizations and site management organizations. The claim here goes beyond complaints that international research is exploitative because the benefits of research are not fairly shared. The more fundamental concern is that the realities of the current economic model of international research effectively prevent affected populations and their governments from influencing the research agenda and organization.[22,23]

Next, consider the dramatic underrepresentation of women's perspectives and interests in research that is not reducible to a problem of unfair distribution of the benefits and burdens of research that could be corrected by increasing the proportion of women enrolled in clinical trials (see Chapter 6). A long-standing problem of no less significance is that the research agenda reflects oppressive social norms that reinforce the view that women are mere "vessels and vectors," rather than persons with their own voice, rights, and interests. Oppression does not merely disempower potential research participants; the lack of female researchers in certain domains also affects the research agenda and priorities. Historian Jessica Martucci[24] has, for instance, shown that the study of breastfeeding practices immensely benefited from the involvement of female researchers. The same argument has been made with respect to pervasive racial prejudices and injustices, which translate into problems in subject selection and in difficulties that major research institutions face, even when they acknowledge their deficiencies, in recruiting and retaining health researchers and bioethicists from diverse, underrepresented, and disadvantaged backgrounds. On these issues, one can only concur with Michael Marmot, "At the end of every scientific paper there is a familiar coda: more research is needed, more research is needed. What, I wondered, if we added a new coda: more action is needed. It need not be discordant with the first" (p. 17).[25]

Finally, there is growing attention to patient-led research (PLR), that is, research projects spontaneously initiated by patients who self-organize in selecting a research question, study design, data collection and analysis method, and dissemination of study results. One of the main arguments in favor of facilitating PLR is that they serve "the individual right to scientific and cultural participation and the common good of a more participatory scientific culture" (p. 218).[26] This right, if there indeed is such a right, cannot be derived from principles of distributive justice but might be tightly connected to a principle of nondomination, which precludes exclusion from certain valuable social practices and presses respect for individuals as knowers, not merely as bodies instrumental for the conduct of research. In addition, by taking the lead in setting the research agenda, patients transform tacit institutional models of what constitutes the "social value" of science and who is entitled to define it.

The recognition of the PLR would correct a salient form of domination, what Miranda Fricker[27] calls an epistemic injustice, that is, a wrong done to someone specifically as a knower. Epistemic injustice primarily reflects a prejudice in the economy of credibility: the wrongful, habitual nonacceptance of an individual's testimonial based on negative stereotypes. Fricker's theory can be readily applied to patients' advocacy organizations' claim that they have been wrongfully excluded from health research and need to be included in the determination of research priorities and design. Through this lens, PLR appears to be a new step for self-advocacy groups, which claim expertise both in theoretical knowledge and experiential, socially situated knowledge.[28] PLR challenges the view that science is a social practice with exclusive authority claims on the legitimate production of generalizable health knowledge. Thus, the problem of participation leads to issues related to the principles of nonoppression and nondomination that will each likely be the focal points of debates in the years to come.

Principles of Justice Beyond Subject Selection

Although many discussions of principles of justice in research focus on subject selection, they have also been deployed to cover other territories, some of which were briefly touched upon above (e.g., selection of knowledge producers). Another important territory is the allocation of financial and nonfinancial resources to health research.[29] Should resources be allocated to health research rather than to other important social goods? How should resources be equitably distributed between multiple valuable and sometimes competing ends (health, social value, economic development, educational opportunity, etc.) and between current and future generations? How should resources be allocated between basic biomedical science, where likely benefits are more long-term, and clinical, public health, and health systems research, where hoped for benefits are more proximate?

In addition, considerations of justice play a central role in choice of the criteria for setting research priorities and in determining what counts as a fair process for making priority decisions within health research. Which health research questions and which causes of burdens of disease should be given priority? Racial and gender discrimination (see, e.g., Chapters 6 and 7).[29] Considerations of compensatory justice often compete with more traditional criteria for resource allocation, such as the potential for the prevention or treatment of diseases that are the most widespread, alter life expectancy negatively, impact our ability to address health issues that afflict the young or than the old or to treat illnesses that cause the most pain and suffering.

Another Route: Developing Theories of Justice in Health Research Contexts

Having examined the principles of justice at play in health research ethics debates, I turn to a different approach. Could *theories* of justice enlighten health research issues? Two reasons motivate my inquiry. First, principles of justice are not stand-alone norms. Their meaning and justification depend upon theories of justice, broadly understood as systematic articulations of a conception of justice. For example, the discussion on the recognition and regulation of PLR has led some to propose a "new social contract" for research (p. 218).[26] However, the framework of the social contract is perhaps not the most helpful way to justify the research enterprise and its oversight. PLR could be grounded in competing theories of justice that have no recourse to ideas of the social contract. Similarly, debates over an alleged obligation to participate in research would benefit from a more systematic articulation of the theories of justice underlying research. Some theories of justice have the potential to assign responsibilities for conducting and funding research, and provide precise guidance for setting priorities. Finally, theories of justice can certainly assist in identifying and addressing the most pressing justice issues, beyond the distribution/oppression/domination distinctions that intervene in debates about principles of justice.

Second, extant attempts to use theories of justice as the starting point for an inquiry into research ethics are either incomplete because they are focused on a limited territory (e.g., international clinical trials[30,31] or health systems research[32]), or unsatisfactory because their methodological approach is problematic. The latter critique can be leveraged against David Buchanan and Franklin Miller.[29] These authors compare the specific and different ramifications of several theories of justice in health research contexts, and wrongly assume that those theories are directly relevant to health research contexts (see my comments on Rawls below). In order to fill this gap and supplement approaches based on principles of justice, I explore a different approach that draws on contemporary debates in political philosophy on justice theory. Rather than advocating a particular theory of justice, my goal is to circumscribe the main features of theories of justice that would be well-positioned to be expanded and specified to advance debates over the fullest range of issues in health research contexts. To do this I proceed in three steps. I first explore the site of theories of justice (i.e., the kinds of objects that are appropriately governed by the principles of justice specified by a theory). I next turn to the scope of theories of justice (i.e., the range of agents to whom considerations of justice apply). I finish by turning to the goals of theories of justice (i.e., the job a theory of justice is supposed to accomplish).

The Site of Theories of Justice

The site of justice refers to the kinds of objects that a theory of justice is designed to cover.[33] These can include, for example, the actions or character of individuals, private interactions between individuals, nonprofit or for-profit private associations (e.g., universities, nongovernmental organizations, private foundations, business firms, labor unions, religious institutions, private hospitals), and basic social, economic, and political institutions.

Theories of justice always select one or several related objects as the site of justice. This is why they often acknowledge that the remaining territories, which are not of significance to their projects, require theories of justice of their own. Major theories of justice identify different sites of justice, not all of which fit well with health research as an enterprise that involves institutions, associations, and individuals. Here, my focus is on alternative ways to characterize the site of *social* justice considering the sharp contrast between John Rawls's and Norman Daniels's theories on the one hand and Madison Powers's and Ruth Faden's theory on the other.

The starting point of any contemporary theory of social justice is the work of Rawls. In his words, "the primary subject of [social] justice is the basic structure of society" (p. 7).[34] What Rawls means by the basic structure of society is disputable but arguably he is interested in the most basic rules of social cooperation for mutual advantage that govern the social, economic, and political institutions that have the deepest and most pervasive impact on people's lives. Examples include basic constitutional entitlements (fundamental liberties and rights), rules that secure fair equality of opportunity in employment and education beyond nondiscrimination based on race, gender, or religion, and the most general rules that constrain the distribution of income and wealth, such as the tax system and inheritance laws.

Does a Rawlsian understanding of social justice directly cover health research institutions and practices? The short answer is no. The principles that govern the basic structure do not directly apply to nonbasic public institutions (e.g., public research institutions), private associations (e.g., pharmaceutical companies), or individuals' actions (e.g., investigators, citizens as potential research subjects). Moreover, the principles of justice that govern these territories are not derivable from the principles of social justice. Hence, Rawls's own theory has the potential to offer only limited guidance for justice issues in health research. What a Rawlsian perspective can directly offer is a critique of background conditions under which health research takes place, including general laws that permit the accumulation of wealth, creating deep inequalities that impact health and the capacity to invest in research or influence its agenda.

Can a Rawlsian theory of justice be modified so as to cover health research? Our best chance is to examine Daniels's attempt to expand Rawls's theory of justice to health contexts.[1-2] Daniels is acutely aware that Rawls's characterization of the site of justice raises a serious obstacle for his project when he notes that, "The most promising strategy for extending Rawls's theory simply includes health-care institutions and practices among the basic institutions involved in providing for fair equality of opportunity" (p. 45).[1] The argument for the inclusion of health-care institutions to broaden the site of justice is that Rawls erroneously adopts a simplified idealizing assumption that individuals are "normal, active, and fully cooperating members of society over the course of a complete life" (p. 302).[34] Once we endorse a more realistic assumption, Daniels argues that shortfalls from normal functioning due to illness negatively impact the opportunity range of at least some people. Therefore, the scope of application of the principle of fair equality of opportunity should not be restricted to employment and education (as Rawls believed). A more capacious account of opportunity is needed. Daniels argues that universal access to reasonable care is necessary (though not sufficient) to secure the health needs of individuals. In recent years, Daniels has extended his account beyond health care to cover other pathways through which individuals' and populations' health needs are met. His focus is now on a broader range of "socially controllable factors that affect population health and its distribution" (p. 30).[2]

The important point here is that the extension of Rawls's theory to health care requires a substantial modification of that theory, but still, in its present form, Daniels's theory does not explicitly cover health research. One promising way to extend Daniels's theory has been explored by Bridget Pratt and colleagues.[31] They persuasively argue that if Daniels conceives the goal of health care to be providing optimal care to everyone, then health research is necessary. Daniels's egalitarian and maximizing goal has implications in terms of the range of health research that can be supported on the basis of his theory compared to alternative views. Those who deny that health care needs to be optimal in any sense of the term will give support to a much narrower range of health research.[35,36] Those who set a higher standard of what counts as optimal health will lend support to a wider range of health research.[4]

In contrast to Rawls's view and Daniels's amended Rawlsian approach, some theories endorse from the outset a broader understanding of the subject matter of social justice and are thereby equipped to cover a broader range of issues in health research. For instance, Powers and Faden write that, "questions of justice emerge from the operation of the totality of social institutions, practices, and policies that both independently and in combination have the potential for profound and pervasive impact on human wellbeing in all of its essential aspects" (p. 5).[3] The purview of their theory is not limited to basic social, economic, and political institutions, or even to health care and public health institutions. It includes any institution and nonprofit or for-profit private association involved in practices that have a profound and pervasive impact on individuals' well-being.

Powers and Faden work with a multidimensional understanding of well-being that encompasses six core elements that are necessary for a decent human life: health, cognition, personal security, personal attachments, the enjoyment of equal respect of others, and self-determination. Central to their theory is the idea of unjust disadvantage. A person is unjustly disadvantaged if he or she suffers deprivation in at least one of these elements of well-being because social arrangements put others in a superior position. It is especially urgent to alter these social arrangements if they create or reinforce patterns of systematic disadvantage that compound the effects of various deprivations on some individuals or groups.

Powers and Faden's theory has the potential to offer particular insights on justice in health research. One reason is that health research and its findings can have a profound and pervasive impact on health through a variety of social institutions and practices. But the reach of health research extends as well to several other core dimensions of well-being, such as personal security, reasoning capacities, personal emotional attachments, respect by others, and self-determination.

For example, health research can identify particularly important threats to well-being such as the potential life-long impact of deprivation in early childhood. But the impact of early childhood deprivation reaches other dimensions of well-being. They may cause deficiencies in cognitive development, undermine the ability to form emotional attachment to others, and ultimately prevent one from leading a life that is, in its broad contours, self-determining.

Because well-being is a multidimensional concept and because deficiencies in health status are often (but not always) causally linked to deficiencies in other dimensions of well-being, health research needs to track the impact of health interventions and policies on all relevant dimensions of well-being. Besides its role in tracking well-being, health research also has the potential to further the dimensions of well-being irreducible to health. For example, research on reproductive policies may identify means that make it easier for people to control whether and with whom they become parents, and thereby enhance self-determination and attachment. Investment in health research can further personal security, particularly for women, by, for example, supporting new technologies that women can use to prevent sexually transmitted infections or pregnancy without dependence on the cooperation of abusive partners.

A downside of this theory is "mission creep": it might unduly extend the responsibilities of health institutions (and therefore their already overwhelmed agents) to domains traditionally under the purview of other institutions. Note, however, that it also goes the other way round: this theory entails that institutions usually in charge of other elements of well-being, such as personal security, have overlapping responsibilities with health institutions. Although this objection is fair, it is not fatal. Any theory of justice not committed to artificially separate "spheres" of justice has to explain how responsibilities for protecting and promoting well-being have to be socially distributed in a manner that is efficient, procedurally, and substantially fair, psychologically acceptable to situated and bounded agents, culturally appropriate, and politically feasible. This is certainly an area for future investigation that would benefit from localized discussions, rather than purely theoretical debates on fairness in the allocation of responsibilities that lack the desirable level of granularity.

To conclude, how the site of justice is characterized within a theory has strong implications with respect to the range of issues a theory can address in health research contexts and the conceptual tools it can deploy.

The Scope of Theories of Justice

Marmot[25] provides staggering descriptions of health inequalities between and within countries. Take life-expectancy at birth. He cites the 2012 WHO data showing that it has a spread from forty-six years in Sierra Leone to eighty-four in Japan.[37] But Marmot notes that in wealthy countries the social gradient of health (i.e., the linking of social position with health) is also arresting: life expectancy varies by twenty years for men in certain areas of Baltimore and Glasgow.[25]

While research identifies health disparities, it does not answer the normative question: Is improving the lot of the disadvantaged at home as morally significant as the welfare of the disadvantaged abroad, who might be doing worse in absolute terms? There is no easy answer, and in particular, the defenders of "global health" should not beg the question. If "global health" is primarily construed in terms of the scope of the problems we are facing (e.g., infectious diseases, poverty-related ill health), and not in terms of their location (i.e., beyond the borders of high-income countries), then its empirical and normative focus could include domestic inequalities as well as international ones.[38,39] Here, philosophical debates on the scope of justice might prove useful for clarifying our options and their justification. The scope of justice "refers to the range of persons who have claims upon and responsibilities to each other arising from considerations of justice" (p. 232).[33] Are obligations of justice limited to members of a particular country? If obligations of justice extend beyond national borders, is their content thinner and their strength weaker than in the domestic arena? Three families of theories offer various answers to these questions.

Strong "statist" theories claim that obligations of justice arise only within nation-states. A variety of reasons are invoked in support of that claim. Thomas Nagel, for instance, has argued for a distinctively political conception of justice according to which the scope and the site of justice are coextensive.[40] Obligations of justice arise between citizens of democratic states who are subject to coercive laws that affect their life prospects. As no global authority exerts a similar type of legal coercion, citizens of affluent countries and their states do not owe any obligation of justice to the global poor. What they owe them is a humanitarian duty of assistance that arises because of the absolute level of need of some populations that the affluent are in a position to help. Hence, even if there are genuine moral duties of assistance, these have a strict and low cut-off point: the satisfaction of basic needs rather than the higher standards set of well-being, human flourishing, or, as Marmot puts it, the goal of bringing the health indicators of everybody to match the top fifth of the best-off populations.[25] With respect to health research funding, strong statists would deny that there is any obligation of justice to allocate part of the research fund of affluent states to researching diseases and conditions that do not affect their own citizens. Alternatively, they might argue that moral duties of assistance might support the allocation of some research funding to causes (whatever those are) of severe burdens of disease in parts of the world where there is substantial suffering and need, or that improving the health of disadvantaged populations is instrumentally justified to promote domestic health and national security.

At the other end of the spectrum, some authors defend cosmopolitan theories of justice that do not restrict obligations of justice to members of a particular society but instead take the view that national boundaries are irrelevant to duties and claims of justice.[41] Several strategies are open to cosmopolitans.[42] They may argue that affluent nations impose on the global poor an international order in ways that make their transactions substantially nonvoluntary, if not outright coercive. Another strategy is to argue that the current distribution of wealth and power is due to past wrongs that need to be rectified and to present forms of structural injustice in the design of global institutions and forms of exchange from which affluent nations wrongfully benefit. A third strategy is to argue for cosmopolitanism directly from people's common humanity that provides them all with the same bundle of rights claims.

Whatever strategy is adopted, for cosmopolitans the current global distribution of wealth and power is unjust. Cosmopolitan reasoning directly challenges the view that states and private funders should give priority to the health research needs of the members of their society. It provides a strong theoretical rationale for claiming that inequalities of the magnitude of the "10/ 90 gap" (i.e., the claim that 10 percent of worldwide expenditure on clinical research is allocated to health issues that affect 90 percent of the world's population[43]) is unjust and that research resources should be allocated in ways that track the global burden of disease, and not a national one. Nonetheless, strong differences among cosmopolitan views persist. Depending on their determination of the factors that are believed to trigger duties of justice, each theory provides a rationale for health research funding, interventions, and priorities that addresses health inequalities that have a specific source (e.g., inequalities caused by past wrongs, including domestic wrongs due to pervasive racial or class-based discrimination).

Hybrid theorists reject both strong statism and cosmopolitanism.[2,44,45] They agree with cosmopolitans about basic universal rights claims and the moral arbitrariness of restricting duties of justice to cocitizens. But they also argue that nation-states have special obligations toward their own citizens and/or residents that go beyond their global obligations of justice to all. These theories therefore provide various arguments for a range of just priority-setting criteria in allocating health research funds that do not simply track the global burden of disease and might have the theoretical space to accommodate the view that reducing the domestic social gradient of health is a moral imperative of equal significance. In addition, hybrid theories would require the development of specific international agencies and rule-making bodies that would channel and fairly distribute resources, as well as regulate international research.[2]

To sum up, the scope of justice delineates the obligations of justice due to non-co-nationals and can play a role in specifying the normative goals of "global health" and research to address health inequalities. Importantly, the scope of justice does not cover all moral duties and concerns (e.g., humanitarian assistance). Solidarity, too, should inform our moral sensibility to justice and help us recognize, beyond the realm of legitimate rights claims, the significance of mutual interdependence, care, and concern, and motivate us to "stand up beside" others, be they close-by or far away.[46,47]

The Goals of Theories of Justice

In this last section, I will contrast two possible goals of a theory of justice, ideal and nonideal theorizing, which bear on the methods used to approach justice problems in health research. A theory of justice might develop a conception of a perfectly just state of affairs (e.g., at the interpersonal or societal level) and of the set of more requirements that are jointly necessary and sufficient to govern it. This is what Rawls calls "ideal theory" (pp. 8–9).[34] He argues that ideal theory has conceptual and normative priority over finding out what is normatively required to address urgent real-world injustices. A vision of an ideally just society offers tools for evaluating the justness of the situation we now face. However, to become more action-guiding in the actual world, where unjust inequalities are part of the background, additional considerations would be needed. These considerations would move us closer to the perfectly just society that the theory identifies and defends. The latter point is important, since my aim is not to argue that ideal theory should be avoided in health research ethics. Aspirational moral, social, and political values are indispensable. The point is that ideal theory has to be carefully supplemented by empirical, theoretical, political, and normative considerations that bridge the gap between the ideal and the actual.

In contrast to ideal theories, some theories set themselves the task of diagnosing and treating the most pressing injustices that occur in real-world settings. These "nonideal" theories approach justice issues by comparing different "feasible" social and institutional arrangements that would enable either reducing injustices or advancing justice.[48] To achieve these ends, nonideal theorists mobilize the best scientific understanding of human behavior and its motivation, of the functioning of institutions and social practices, and of the actual causal structure of the natural and social world. They concede neither a conceptual nor a normative priority to the vision of a perfectly just society over the task of identifying and addressing real-world injustices. However, there is room for debate as to whether pure nonideal theory is even possible or whether the introduction of some idealizing assumptions in modeling societies and institutions is unavoidable and should be acknowledged (see below).

The nonideal/ideal theory debate can shed light on some heated debates in research ethics, such as the moral obligation to participate in health research. Rosamond Rhodes has made an ideal theory argument in favor of the obligation to participate in research.[49] Social contract theories purport to establish the legitimacy of political authority and the moral obligations of citizens of a state who give consent to a mutually beneficial and enforceable hypothetical contract. According to Rhodes, any reasonable person should accept an obligation to periodic service as a research subject because general cooperation is necessary to advance medical science from which all parties stand to benefit through improved medical care. Refraining from participation would constitute unjust free-riding, a breach of "biological citizenship," as anthropologists would put it.

This argument determines research participation obligations assuming that individuals live in a society that is in all other respects just. Society's politically enforceable moral norms derive from a hypothetical contract that individuals comply with. Now, pressed as to whether she *actually* defends a legal or even an all-things-considered moral obligation to participate in research, Rhodes responds in the negative:

> My argument is about justice in the allocation of research risks and burdens in the context of a reasonable expectation to have a share in the rewards. In the U.S. today, in numerous explicit and veiled ways, medical resources are not distributed in accordance with justice. So long as the benefits of research are unjustly allocated here, we lack the justification for allocating the risks and burdens of research based on equality. (p. W17)[50]

Given that background justice conditions necessary to ground a universal obligation to participate in research are not satisfied in the United States, it is unclear how much Rhodes's argument from ideal theory contributes to a morally significant discussion in research ethics since it lacks bridge arguments for meaningful implementation of the view. What concrete actions and policies would move us closer to conditions for the ideal allocation of the burden of research?

In contrast, consider another proposal in defense of a justice-based obligation of patients to contribute to the production of medical knowledge.[44] Here, the main objective is to build an ethical framework for a way of reorganizing health-care systems that would not rely on the current distinction between clinical research and clinical practice inherited from the US National Commission's *Belmont Report*.[6,51] In "learning healthcare systems" (LHS), research and practice would be continuously integrated into knowledge development and application in health-care delivery, rather than segregated.[52,53] LHS raise fundamental questions: through what mechanisms should learning activities be ethically regulated, no matter where they fall along the research-practice continuum, and why? What are the ethical obligations of health-care providers and patients in LHS? Faden and colleagues argue that patients have an obligation to participate in certain limited learning activities based on norms of common purpose and reciprocity:

> [Some] learning activities—such as participation in a registry, reviews of deidentified medical records, and being interviewed by health care staff to better improve the patient care experience—are likely to

be instances in which patients do have an obligation to participate, *assuming* that the activities have a *reasonable likelihood* of improving health care quality and that appropriate data security protections are in place. *These conditions are probably met currently* in integrated health care systems that have invested in secure electronic health records and have mechanisms in place to adjust local norms of care in direct response to the result of learning activities. (*emphasis* added) (p. S23)[52]

Although the authors do not present their work as a case study in nonideal theory, it embodies some of its characteristics. They make no idealizing assumption about the virtues of individuals or the justice of society in general; they make limited idealizing assumptions about how the improved health-care system would function, but carefully evaluate the distance between what currently obtains in existing integrated health-care systems and what the model demands. Their model is built in sufficient proximity with the real world so as to enable the representation of a realistic transformation of current systems, without losing its normative bite.

Conclusion

In this chapter I have discussed the role that principles of justice have so far played in debates on the ethics of health research. My claim is that the move from the *Belmont Report* that inspired a protective approach to health research to an approach stressing the access to the potential benefits of research should not be interpreted as the endorsement of a conception of justice solely concerned with respect for autonomous decisions of individuals. On the contrary, the movement in favor of increased access to the opportunity to participate in health research goes hand in hand with a more expansive conception of the principles of justice that ought to govern research. These principles include a requirement of nonoppression and nondomination, in addition to the fair distribution of the benefits and burdens of research among individuals and groups. They have informed and continue to feed the debate on the ethics of health research.

Although traditionally, justice issues in health research have been discussed through the lens of principles of justice, I argue in this chapter for an alternative approach. In my view, theories of justice developed in political philosophy or biomedical and public health ethics need to be expanded and specified to provide coherent approaches to the fullest range of health research justice issues. Each theory of justice has its own strength and weaknesses, and my goal was not to argue in favor of one of them. Rather, I delineated the main features of these theories that would enable them to be responsive to the distinctively justice-related challenges of the contemporary research enterprise.

Notes

1. Daniels N. *Just Health Care*. Cambridge, England: Cambridge University Press; 1985.
2. Daniels N. *Just Health: Meeting Health Needs Fairly*. New York, NY: Cambridge University Press; 2008.
3. Powers M, Faden R. *Social Justice: The Moral Foundations of Public Health and Health Policy*. New York, NY: Oxford University Press; 2006.
4. Ruger JP. *Health and Social Justice*. New York, NY: Oxford University Press; 2009.
5. Venkatapuram S. *Health Justice: An Argument from the Capabilities Approach*. Oxford, England: Wiley; 2013.
6. National Commission for the Protection of Human Subjects of Biomedical and Behavioral Research. The Belmont Report: Ethical principles and guidelines for the protection of human subjects of research. *Federal Register*. 1979;44(76):23192–23197.
7. McCarthy CR. The evolving story of justice in federal research policy. In: Kahn JP, Mastroianni AC, Sugarman J, eds. *Beyond Consent: Seeking Justice in Research*. New York, NY: Oxford University Press; 1998:11–31.
8. Baker R. *Before Bioethics: A History of American Medical Ethics from the Colonial Period to the Bioethics Revolution*. New York, NY: Oxford University Press; 2013.
9. Powers M. Theories of justice in the context of research. In: Kahn JP, Mastroianni AC, Sugarman J, eds. *Beyond Consent: Seeking Justice in Research*. New York, NY: Oxford University Press; 1998:147–165.
10. Engelhardt HT Jr. *The Foundations of Bioethics*. New York, NY: Oxford University Press; 1986.
11. Epstein RA. Defanging IRBs: replacing coercion with information. *Northwestern University Law Review*. 2007;101(1):735–748.
12. Code of Federal Regulations, Title 45, Public Welfare Department of Health and Human Services, Part 46; 1981.
13. Mastroianni AC, Kahn J. Swinging on the pendulum: shifting views of justice in human subjects research. *Hastings Center Report*. 2001;31(3):21–28.
14. Epstein, S. *Inclusion: The Politics of Difference in Medical Research*. Chicago, IL: University of Chicago Press; 2007.
15. Wertheimer A. *Rethinking the Ethics of Clinical Research: Widening the Lens*. New York, NY: Oxford University Press; 2010.
16. Wertheimer A. The obligations of researchers amidst injustice or deprivation. In: Millum J, Emanuel EJ, eds. *Global Justice and Bioethics*. New York, NY: Oxford University Press; 2012:279–304.

17. Wenner DM. The social value of knowledge and international clinical research. *Developing World Bioethics.* 2015;15(2):76–84.

18. Young IM. *Justice and the Politics of Difference.* Princeton, NJ: Princeton University Press; 1990.

19. Pettit P. *On the People's Terms: A Republican Theory and Model of Democracy.* Cambridge, MA: Cambridge University Press; 2012.

20. Lovett F. *A General Theory of Domination and Justice.* New York, NY: Oxford University Press; 2010.

21. Bachvarova M. Non-domination's role in the theorizing of global justice. *Journal of Global Ethics.* 2013;9(2):173–185.

22. Petryna A. *When Experiments Travel: Clinical Trials and the Global Search for Human Subjects.* Princeton, NJ: Princeton University Press; 2007.

23. Mitra AG. A social connection model for international clinical research. *American Journal of Bioethics.* 2013;13(3):W1–W2.

24. Martucci J. *Back to the Breast: Natural Motherhood and Breastfeeding in America.* Chicago, IL: University of Chicago Press; 2015.

25. Marmot M. *The Health Gap: The Challenge of an Unequal World.* London, England: Bloomsbury; 2015.

26. Vayena E, Brownsword R, Edwards SJ, et al. Research led by participants: a new social contract for a new kind of research. *Journal of Medical Ethics.* 2016;42(4):216–219. doi:10.1136/medethics-2015-102663.

27. Fricker M. *Epistemic Injustice: Power and the Ethics of Knowing.* Oxford, England: Oxford University Press; 2007.

28. Schicktanz S. The ethical legitimacy of patient organizations' involvement in politics and knowledge production: epistemic justice as a conceptual basis. In: Wehling P, Viehöver W, Koenen S, eds. *The Public Shaping of Medical Research: Patient Associations, Health Movements and Biomedicine.* New York, NY: Routledge; 2015:246–264.

29. Buchanan D, Miller FG. Justice in research on human subjects. In: Rhodes R, Battin M, Silvers A, eds. *Medicine and Social Justice: Essays on the Distribution of Health Care.* New York, NY: Oxford University Press; 2012:445–460.

30. London AJ. Justice and the human development approach to international research. *Hastings Center Report.* 2005;35(1):24–37.

31. Pratt B, Zion D, Loff B. Evaluating the capacity of theories of justice to serve as a justice framework for international clinical research. *American Journal of Bioethics.* 2012;12(11):30–41. doi:10.1080/15265161.2012.719261.

32. Pratt B, Hyder AA. Global justice and health systems research in low- and middle-income countries. *Journal of Law, Medicine & Ethics.* 2015;43(1):143–161.

33. Abizadeh A. Cooperation, pervasive impact, and coercion: on the scope (not site) of distributive justice. *Philosophy & Public Affairs.* 2007;35(4):318–358.

34. Rawls J. *A Theory of Justice.* Cambridge, MA: Harvard University Press; 1971.

35. Jonas H. Philosophical reflections on experimenting with human subjects. *Daedalus.* 1969;98(2):219–247.

36. Callahan D. *What Price Better Health? Hazards of the Research Imperative.* Berkeley, CA: University of California Press; 2003.

37. World Health Organization. Global Health Observatory data repository: Life expectancy data by country. http://apps.who.int/gho/data/node.main.688. Cited in: Marmot M. *The Health Gap: The Challenge of an Unequal World.* London, England: Bloomsbury; 2015.

38. Koplan JP, Bond TC, Merson MH, et al. Towards a common definition of global health. *Lancet.* 2009;373(9679):1993–1995. doi: 10.1016/S0140-6736(09)60332-9.

39. Hunter D, Dawson AJ. Is there a need for global health ethics? For and against. In: Benatar S, Brock G, eds. *Global Health and Global Health Ethics.* Cambridge, England: Cambridge University Press; 2011:77–88.

40. Nagel T. The problem of global justice. *Philosophy & Public Affairs.* 2005;33(2):113–147.

41. Pogge T. *World Poverty and Human Rights: Cosmopolitan Responsibilities and Reforms.* Cambridge, England: Polity Press; 2002.

42. Powers M. Social justice. In: Jennings B, ed. *Encyclopedia of Bioethics.* 4th ed. New York, NY: Macmillan Publishing Company; 2014:2966–2973.

43. Global Forum for Health Research. The 10/90 report on health research 2003–2004. Geneva, Switzerland: Global Forum for Health Research; 2004. http://announcementsfiles.cohred.org/gfhr_pub/assoc/s14789e/s14789e.pdf. Accessed December 4, 2017.

44. Miller D. *National Responsibility and Global Justice.* New York, NY: Oxford University Press; 2007.

45. Ruger JP. Good medical ethics, justice and provincial globalism. *Journal of Medical Ethics.* 2015;41(1):103–106.

46. Ijsselmuiden CB, Kass NE, Sewankambo KN, Lavery JV. Evolving values in ethics and global health research. *Global Public Health.* 2010;5(2):154–163.

47. Jennings B, Dawson A. Solidarity in the moral imagination of bioethics. *Hastings Center Report.* 2015;45(5):31–38.

48. Sreenivasan G. Non-ideal theory: a taxonomy with illustration. In: Millum J, Emanuel EJ, eds. *Global Justice and Bioethics.* New York, NY: Oxford University Press; 2012:135–152.

49. Rhodes R. Rethinking research ethics. *American Journal of Bioethics.* 2005;5(1):7–28.

50. Rhodes R. Response to commentators on "rethinking research ethics." *American Journal of Bioethics.* 2005;5(1):W15–W18.

51. Beauchamp T, Saghai Y. The historical foundations of the research-practice distinction in bioethics. *Theoretical Medicine and Bioethics.* 2012;33(1):45–56.

52. Faden RR, Kass NE, Goodman SN, Pronovost P, Tunis S, Beauchamp TL. An ethics framework for a learning health care system: a departure from traditional research ethics and clinical ethics. *Hastings Center Report.* 2013;43(S1)S16–S27.

53. Kass NE, Faden RR, Goodman SN, Pronovost P, Tunis S, Beauchamp TL. The research-treatment distinction: a problematic approach for determining which activities should have ethical oversight. *Hastings Center Report.* 2013;43(S1):S4–S15.

12 PURSUING JUSTICE IN RESEARCH

Jeffrey P. Kahn
Anna C. Mastroianni
Jeremy Sugarman

The chapters in this volume examine how the concept of justice has been and should be applied to particular research settings and groups of research participants. Those discussions are multifaceted and do not simply recapitulate the traditional explicit concerns about justice in research that are recognized in regulations (e.g., considerations of subject selection by investigators and institutional review boards (IRBs)[1] in the United States). While those and other considerations of distributive justice are critical, such a narrow application of justice is incomplete.[2]

Policies in the United States dating to the 1970s largely tasked IRBs with addressing justice concerns, but the reality today is that those issues arise in a multitude of arenas and involve a variety of decision-makers at differing points in the research process. Thus, the locus of decision-making for justice issues arising in research must be recognized as no longer solely that of IRBs. Concerns about justice, in fact, permeate the research process—from decisions about research priorities and formulation of research questions, to the design and conduct of research, and the dissemination of research findings. Yet attention to considerations of justice in those diverse contexts has either been lacking or largely implicit, with negative implications for individuals, populations, and the research enterprise generally, as illustrated through the examinations in each of the chapters of this book. A comprehensive understanding therefore involves an understanding of how justice affects and is impacted at each decision point in the research process. Below we highlight some of the justice-related issues arising through the research process and then provide our suggestions to ensure that justice is implemented throughout it.

Implementing Justice in Research

Decision-makers at different points in potential research pathways can influence whether and which issues of justice are relevant to particular areas of research. Moreover, many of their decisions, and the justice issues related to them, are influenced by concerns that fall outside typical scientific design considerations. As documented in a number of chapters in this volume, historical and dominant social forces, for example, may influence the selection of particular populations for research and the development of specific research priorities. Further, decisions that have implications for justice take place at all levels of the research enterprise, routinely and constantly, consciously or not. To address concerns about justice in research more effectively, it is essential to recognize the decision points and decision-makers in the research pathway and what influences their decision-making.

Each functional step in the development and conduct of research defines a decision point. Those points can include: the origination of a research idea, funding for research, study design, prior review, conduct of research, recruitment and retention of research participants, analyses of data, interpretation of findings, dissemination of results, and obligations to and of those who participated in research and their communities. Each of those aspects of research are performed and influenced by various individuals and groups that include: researchers and scientists, federal and state legislative bodies and executive branch agencies and officials, governmental and organizational scientific advisory councils, research foundations, advocacy groups, pharmaceutical and biotechnology companies, research funding review committees, educational and noneducational institutions in which research is performed, IRBs, data monitoring committees, patients and research participants, journal editors, journal peer reviewers, international bodies, and professional organizations. With all that in mind, by following a roughly chronological process through the research pathway, it is possible to examine the types of situations in which concerns about justice become relevant.

Take, for example, a novel research idea, such as a particular mechanism in the development of heart disease, that may be discussed among members of the faculty of a medical school or the staff of a pharmaceutical or biotechnology company. By focusing on this question, another potentially important research focus may be forgone, raising questions about justice.

Research ideas may be the product of scientific curiosity, but they are also as likely to be prompted by funding announcements about research on a particular disease, institutional incentives or rewards, or lobbying from advocacy groups. Regardless, the decision by an individual investigator—whether a university faculty member or staff scientist—to pursue a research idea has implications for the population(s) that will be enrolled in the research and that may potentially benefit from its results.

Funding, however, is obviously necessary before even promising research ideas can be pursued. More research funding means the possibility for research with more and different populations and the opportunity for the inclusion of additional members of particular populations in research. Yet funding determinations reflect a range of previous decisions in the public sector (e.g., National Institutes of Health (NIH)) and private sector (e.g., pharmaceutical and biotechnology companies and private foundations). Those determinations also reflect larger decisions about allocation of resources to biomedical research instead of to other societal goods, such as defense, education, and transportation. At its most basic, when a government makes a decision to spend additional funds on medical research or to cut research expenditures, there are serious implications for the quantity of research that can be performed, as well as the range of research ideas that can be examined.

Within the private sector, research and development costs must be balanced against other corporate costs, including personnel, manufacturing, and marketing costs. Decisions about overall funding can also be influenced by advocacy efforts of those receiving research support, such as research institutions, and those who stand to realize the potential benefit of the results of research, such as patient-advocacy groups. Thus, a cascade occurs through the system that raises questions about distributive justice, since funding is|a finite resource and research can only be practicably carried out in relatively small groups of people. Not only does that mean that particular populations can be potentially burdened, or conversely receive direct immediate benefits from participation in research, it also means that the potential meaningfulness of research results within a population in which an intervention was not evaluated is affected.

Whatever the level of research funding, whether it be in the public or private sector, decisions about research priorities raise obvious justice considerations. Providing financial incentives, or removing disincentives, can work to directly or indirectly ensure a fairer distribution of limited resources. For instance, legislators may assert their spending authority by earmarking resources for research on a particular disease or condition, or even a specific population.[3] Pharmaceutical and biotechnology companies make decisions about research and development with potential markets in mind, so may concentrate on diseases with high or increasing prevalence, and in the process may exclude those with less-prevalent conditions. That is, eventual success in the marketplace is an essential driver of priority-setting in the private sector. Policymakers have developed some counterweights in response to this tendency, including incentives for orphan drug development to encourage product development for low prevalence (i.e., small market) diseases. Those policies serve to encourage justice in drug development by subsidizing the cost of research and development, and providing a financial incentive to pharmaceutical companies through provisions for longer periods of market exclusivity.

Private research foundations also make decisions with justice implications for the research enterprise. They make decisions consistent with their stated missions, whether they be disease-specific (e.g., the American Cancer Society, the American Heart Association) or issue-specific (e.g., the Ford Foundation's interest in specific international settings).

Decisions by review groups of various types, whether peer review groups in the traditional NIH–style councils or by those within private entities, can have justice implications. For instance, with only a small proportion of research applications funded in a given year, decisions favoring research on one disease or population versus another can have a significant impact. While some explicit consideration has been given to "gender and minority representation" in US government-sponsored research since the 1990s, the extent to which such considerations ultimately ensure justice is a work in progress,[4,5] and, importantly, the degree to which they are incorporated in other settings is unclear.

Once funded, individual research projects typically undergo prospective review by an IRB. At this point, justice plays a role in determining how subjects should be selected, and the intervention subjects should receive once selected and appropriately enrolled. The practical aspects of carrying out research, from recruitment and retention of subjects to the conditions under which participation ensues, also have implications for justice. For example, the process employed in choosing individual subjects must be fair.

Access to participation in research is affected not only by the criteria by which eligibility is determined, but also by the mechanisms used to recruit subjects. For example, while web or social media-based recruitment may be effective,[6] such approaches may also skew access toward a particular population, thereby introducing potential concerns about justice. Even recruitment through more traditional means, such as venue-based approaches, can introduce justice considerations. That is, particular modes of recruitment may be more or less accessible to particular segments of the potential subject population. Community engagement, discussed in this volume, is one attempt to address justice in recruitment and other areas throughout research pathways.

Once research has been carried out, the reporting, analysis, and dissemination of results are critical steps between research and its applications. Decisions about how widely research results are reported typically lie in the hands of investigators and often the sponsors of research. Peer reviewers and journal editors then make decisions about which research is worthy of publication. In the most prestigious journals, editors may also wield considerable influence through editorials about research findings or conduct (for example, an editorial discussion of the ethics of AZT trials for vertical transmission of HIV in Africa[7]). Subsequently, professional opinion may be shaped and popular media may disseminate this information to the public and to policymakers. In turn, this may have significant influence on establishing future research priorities, including the development of future research questions and the populations in which they will be explored.

The forgoing are but a sampling of points in research pathways that do, or should, implicate justice considerations: There exists a web of decisions and decision-makers spanning all aspects of the research pathway. Awareness of this complex web is crucial for understanding the far-reaching scope of justice in research.

Seeking Justice in Research

Given the complexities and interdependencies briefly described above, we propose the following for consideration in the implementation of justice throughout the research enterprise. These suggestions emanate from considering in aggregate the analyses of cases and experiences offered in this volume.

First, comprehensive attention to justice is of fundamental importance to building and maintaining trust in the research enterprise. Without trust, research with human subjects would be much more difficult since the large reservoir of trust on the part of subjects undoubtedly plays an important role in their willingness to participate.[8] Without attention to justice it is difficult to maintain, let alone build, trust and it is quite likely that existing trust will be eroded.

Second, justice in research requires recognition and attention at every level of the decision-making process. Considerations of justice at each decision point must be conscious and explicit, or there is the risk that justice may be overlooked, as the contributors to this volume make clear. Routine mechanisms to ensure accountability of decision-makers and transparency of decision-making could likely do much to contribute to fairness.

Third, decisions are made throughout the research process by a wide variety of actors. The composition of decision-making groups can be tremendously influential at each level. Do the decision-makers as a group represent diverse perspectives and experiences? Further, decisions are made largely without coordination with others who are involved in different aspects of the research enterprise, and the research enterprise has no mechanism by which to coordinate this decision-making. That lack of coordination undermines accountability for the effects of decisions. Whatever coordination exists is also influenced by individuals and groups outside those directly involved in the research, such as advocates. That is not to say that each decision point related to justice is totally isolated from every other. The structure of the research process is such that decisions affecting justice that are overlooked or misguided at one point in the process might be recognized at other points. The problem is that there is no mechanism for ensuring that such perceived missteps will be caught and addressed. It is therefore incumbent upon each actor in the research process to recognize and attend to justice.

Fourth, biases and incentives influencing perceptions of justice in research need to be explicitly acknowledged and disclosed. Decision-makers act in response to the influences, incentives, and biases particular to their situations; decisions are not made in a vacuum. The incentives and perspectives those decision-makers bring to the process, including conflicts of interest and individual agendas, have a clear impact on whether justice in research is served. If decision-makers are explicit about such conflicts and biases, it is more likely that the implications on their actions will be considered.

Fifth, it is essential to incorporate a diversity of views and participation (e.g., genders, underrepresented groups, patients, advocates for diseases, medical conditions, and populations) at each decision-making point in the research process. The participation of subjects—the historically excluded "other" half of the research enterprise—in the decision-making process might make it more likely to meet the demands of justice, avoiding exploitation of some populations as well as the neglect of others. This could include representation and participation in existing advisory and oversight bodies in the research process, as well as other groups that formulate and direct research agendas.[9,10]

Sixth, while pursuit of science should be the basis for doing research, it must be recognized that there are many influences on the determination of what constitutes a relevant scientific question. Values are implicit and inherent at every level of the decision-making process, so it is unrealistic and descriptively false to claim that research is value-free. On this view, claims about science and scientific merit implicate justice. We must realize that evaluation of research involves much more than how any individual investigator thinks about sufficient scientific merit of a particular research area or set of research questions.

Conclusion

Concerns about justice arise at virtually every step along the research pathway. While the research process has a chronological arc, parts of the research process lack integration with each other. For instance, the connection between recruitment and retention issues in a single clinical trial, and funding and allocation decisions being wrestled over at the highest levels of government, seem quite disjointed. Attention to justice at each step, however, forces a relevant connection.

The evolution of the regulations for protection of research subjects and their local application has placed the focus of efforts to serve the rights and interests of research subjects on informed consent and determining acceptable levels of risk in research. While critically important, those issues have come to be the beginning and end of practical research ethics. However, this myopic view of how to achieve ethically appropriate research cannot accomplish its goal.

As we have tried to show, justice is not a simple concept. The multiple conceptions of justice pose a challenge to us in finding ways to apply justice throughout the research process. This challenge must be taken up by all involved in research: We must first acknowledge the challenge and, second, rise to meet it. If we do not, we betray the trust that subjects place in the people, institutions, and processes that make up the research enterprise. It is only by looking beyond consent that the full range of ethical issues in research can be understood, and it is only in acting beyond consent that we can truly seek justice in research.

Notes

1. National Commission for the Protection of Human Subjects of Biomedical and Behavioral Research. The Belmont Report: Ethical principles and guidelines for the protection of human subjects of research. *Federal Register.* 1979;44(76):23192–23197.
2. Powers M. Theories of justice in the context of research. In: Kahn JP, Mastroianni AC, Sugarman J, eds. *Beyond Consent: Seeking Justice in Research.* New York, NY: Oxford University Press; 1998:147–165.
3. The 21st Century Cures Act of 2016, Pub L No 114–255, 130 Stat. 1033.
4. Pinn VW, Clayton JA, Begg L, Sass SE. Public partnerships for a vision for women's health research in 2020. *Journal of Women's Health (Larchmont).* 2010;19(9):1603–1607.
5. Fisher JA, Kalbaugh CA. Challenging assumptions about minority participation in US clinical research. *American Journal of Public Health.* 2011;101(12):2217–2222.

6. Center Watch—Clinical Trial Trends Listing Service website. http://www.centerwatch.com. Accessed December 4, 2017.

7. Angell M. The ethics of clinical research in the third world. *New England Journal of Medicine.* 1997;337(12):847–849.

8. Kass NE, Sugarman J, Faden R, Schoch-Spana M. Trust, the fragile foundation of contemporary biomedical research. *Hastings Center Report.* 1996;26(5):25–29.

9. Frank L, Basch E, Selvy JV, et al. The PCORI perspective on patient-centered outcomes research. *JAMA.* 2014;312(15):1513–1514.

10. Cobb EM, Meurer W, Harney D, et al. Patient engagement in neurological clinical trials design: A conference summary. *Clinical and Translational Science.* 2015;8(6):776–778.

INDEX

Numbers followed by n indicate notes.

AAP (American Academy of Pediatrics), 82–83
aboriginal populations, 138
Accelerated Approval program, 43
access to participation in research, 211
ACHRE (Advisory Committee on Human Radiation Experiments), 21–22, 28–29, 75–76
Ackerman, Terrence, 80
acknowledgment or recognition, 141
ACTG 076 study, 18–19
activism, 8
acute confusional states (delirium), 54
acute, emergent illnesses: research in, 37–42
advance directives, 65–66
Advisory Committee on Human Radiation Experiments (ACHRE), 21–22, 28–29, 75–76
AEC (Atomic Energy Commission), 155
Africa, 97, 169–170
African Americans, 113–115
  Henrietta Lacks, 115–119
  racism against, 7, 102–103, 112–134
  research involving, 123–131
    Grimes v. Kennedy Krieger Institute, Inc., 7, 119–123, 129

prison experiments, 156–157
Tuskegee Syphilis Study (Study of Untreated Syphilis in the Negro Male), 3, 7, 15, 23, 78, 113–115, 121, 125, 130–131, 152
women, 102–103
black women, 102–103
AIDS advocacy, 137–138, 190
AIDS research. *See* HIV/AIDS research
AIDS Vaccine Advocacy Coalition (AVAC), 137–138
All of Us Research Program (Precision Medicine Initiative), 128
allocation of resources, 193, 214
Alzheimer disease (AD), 54, 64–66
Alzheimer disease research, 5
  Cooperative Study centers, 60
  current context, 57–59
  future directions, 63
  public perspectives on, 61–62
American Academy of Pediatrics (AAP), 82–83
American Cancer Society, 211
American Heart Association, 211
American Medical Association (AMA), 155
American Psychological Association (APA), 163

androcentrism, 101
animal studies, 93–94
antiretroviral treatment (ART), 96
apology for wrongs, 20–24, 140, 164–165
Aristotle, 4
Arizona State University, 140
ART (antiretroviral treatment), 96
Ashkenazi Jews, 135–136
assurances, 24
Atomic Energy Commission (AEC), 155
atomic research, 159–160
Attica State Penitentiary, 156
automated external defibrillator (AEDs), 38
AVAC (AIDS Vaccine Advocacy
    Coalition), 137–138
azidothymidine (AZT) studies, 172–173

Bad Blood (Jones), 15
Baltimore, Maryland, 198
Banaji, Mahzarin, 124
Bangladesh: RU-486 trials, 175–176
Bartholome, Willliam, 80
Basic Policy, 25
Bayesian approach, 48
Beecher, Henry, 14–15, 55–56
Beeh, 74
Belmont Report (Ethical Principles and
    Guidelines for the Protection of
    Human Subjects of Research)
    (National Commission), 1–2, 7,
    17–18, 25, 28, 78–79, 125–127,
    157, 170–171, 188–189, 202
benefits of participation in research
  acceptable risks and benefits, 61–63
  fair benefits framework, 176–177,
    180–182
  fair distribution of, 2–4, 13–14, 16–20
  historical examination of, 16–20
  nonobvious, 139–140
  post-trial, 18–20, 176–182
  after study completion, 18–20
beriberi research, 154

Best Pharmaceuticals for Children Act
    (BPCA), 83–85
bias, 117, 123–124, 213
  male, 93–94, 101
BiDil®, 124–125, 131
biological citizenship, 201
Biologics Control Act, 77
blacks. See African Americans
Blindspot (Banaji and
    Greenwald), 124
Bonnie, Richard, 57
botulinum toxoid (BT), 161
Bowman, Phillip, 129
BPCA (Best Pharmaceuticals for
    Children Act), 83–85
BRAIN (Brain Research
    through Advancement
    in Neurotechnologies)
    Initiative, 55
Brandt, Allan, 115
Brazil, 169–170
BRCA1 gene, 135–136
BRCA2 gene, 135–136
breast cancer studies, 135
Brody, Baruch, 4–5
Buchanan, David, 194
burdens of research: allocation
    of, 202

CABs (community advisory boards),
    136–137, 144
California, 57, 61
Cambodia: tenofovir PrEP trials in, 136,
    140–141
Camp Desert Rock, 160
Canadian Tri-Council Policy
    Statement, 138
cancer studies
  chemotherapy trials, 46
  current context, 58
  future directions, 44–45
  historical examination of, 42–44

at Jewish Chronic Disease Hospital
(Brooklyn, NY), 3, 15
Phase I trials, 46
capacity, decisional, 64–66
Capron, Alexander (Alex), 15–16, 28–29
captive populations
pediatric research with, 74–75
regulatory protections
applying to, 18
research with, 8–9, 74–75, 152–168
Cardiac Arrhythmia Suppression Trial
(CAST), 44
cardiovascular research, 94–95
Centers for Disease Control and
Prevention (CDC), 139,
172–173
Centers for Medicare and Medicaid
Services (CMS), 45
Central Intelligence Agency (CIA), 121
chemical weapons research, 161
chemotherapy trials, 46
children. *See also* pediatric research
institutionalized, 74
regulatory protections for, 18
therapeutic orphans, 77–78
vulnerability of, 81–82
China, 169–170, 176
Chisolm, Julian, 120
CIOMS (Council for International
Organizations of Medical
Sciences), 172–173, 178–181
Guideline 10, 178–181
citizenship, biological, 201
Clinical and Translational Science
Awards (CTSAs), 102, 138–139
ClinicalTrials.gov, 93
Clinton, Bill, 19, 22–23
Clinton, Hillary, 23–24, 164–165
Code of Federal Regulations, 79n
coercion, 182
cognitive impairment: research in
populations with, 54–71

current context, 57–59
future directions, 63–66
historical review, 55–57
unresolved issues, 59–61
at Willowbrook State School
(Staten Island, NY), 3, 6, 16,
74–75, 82
collaboration, 183–184
Collins, Francis, 93–94
Colom, Alvaro, 24
combat conditions, 161
Common Rule, 25
communities
definition of, 142–143
disease communities, 143
research communities, 143
respect for, 140–141
community advisory boards (CABs),
136–137, 144
Community Advisory Groups, 144
community engagement, 8, 135–151
call for, 137–139
direct, 144–145
forms of, 143–145
future directions, 145–147
Good Participatory Practice
Guidelines (GPP), 137–138
historical view of, 136–145
institutional approaches
to, 138–139
legitimacy of, 142, 147
meaningfulness of, 146–147
moral foundations of, 139–143
post-trial benefits of, 176–182
requirements for, 138–139, 146, 184
strategies of, 136
compensation 10, 178–181
Compensating for Research Injuries
(President's Commission for
the Study of Ethical Problems in
Medicine and Biomedical and
Behavioral Research), 28

compensatory justice, 3, 14, 20–24, 92
confusion
    acute confusional states
        (delirium), 54
    research in populations with, 55–56
consent, 40
    barriers to, 41
    deferred, 37
    exception from informed consent
        (EFIC), 37–42
    surrogate, 61–63
continual reassessment method
    (CRM), 48
contracts, social, 194, 201
convenient and captive populations.
    See also institutionalized
        subjects
    regulatory protections applying to, 18
    research with, 8–9, 74–75, 152–168
Cooperative Study centers, 60
cosmopolitanism, 199–200
Council for International Organizations
    of Medical Sciences (CIOMS),
    172–173, 178–181
CRM (continual reassessment
    method), 48
CTSAs (Clinical and Translational
    Science Awards), 102, 138–139
cultural differences, 101, 182–183

Daniels, Norman, 195–196
data sharing, 20, 119
DD (democratic deliberation), 62
debates over principles of justice,
    188–193
decisional capacity, 64–66
decisional impairment
    decision-makers for decisionally
        impaired subjects, 59–60
    research in populations with, 54–55
        current context, 57–59
        future directions, 63–66

historical review, 55–57
    unresolved issues, 59
decision-making groups, 212–213
Declaration of Helsinki (DoH), 20, 155,
    172, 177–178
deferred consent, 37
defibrillation research, 38
delirium (acute confusional states), 54
dementia research, 54–55, 62
democratic deliberation (DD), 62
Department of Defense, 159–162
Department of Health and Human
    Services (DHHS), 57, 79n, 100,
    115, 126, 156
    regulations governing federally
        funded research, 61, 100
    Secretary's Advisory Committee on
        Human Research Protections
        (SACHRP), 80
    Task Force on Black and Minority
        Health, 126
    Task Force on Research Specific to
        Pregnant and Lactating Women
        (PRGLAC), 100
Department of Health, Education, and
    Welfare (DHEW), 25
    Basic Policy, 25
    Common Rule, 25
    *PHS Policy and Procedure Order #
        129*, 16
    regulations against prison
        research, 156
    Tuskegee Syphilis Study Ad Hoc
        Advisory Panel, 15–17, 21, 115
DES, 101–102
developed countries, 169–170
developing countries, 169–170
Dickert, Neal, 4–5
disease communities, 143
distributive justice, 7–8, 13–14, 17, 208
    arguments for right to participate in
        research, 189–190

in data sharing, 20
fair distribution of risks and benefits,
    2–4, 13–14, 93, 125–126
    for children, 72–73
    historical examination of, 16–20
    after study completion, 18–20, 176–182
    in global research, 170
    historical examination of, 16–20
    in subject selection, 188–189
    and women's participation, 91–92
diversity, 213
domination, 127–128, 190–193
double standards, 9, 173
Drug Importation Act, 77
drug labeling, 72–73, 77–78, 83–84
drug research & development
    Accelerated Approval program, 43
    continual reassessment method
        (CRM), 48
    Fast Track program, 43
    "Guidelines for the Ethical Conduct
        of Studies to Evaluate Drugs in
        Pediatric Populations" (AAP), 82–83
    history of, 76–78
    off-patent, 83
    pediatric, 72–73, 76–78
    Phase I trials, 45–49
    Phase II trials, 45–46
    and pregnancy, 97–98
    Priority Review program, 43
    prison experiments, 155
    race and racism in, 124–125
    sex differences in, 93
    Treatment Investigational New Drug
        (Treatment IND) program, 43
    women's participation in, 97
DuBois, W. E. B., 114

economic development, 169–170
EFIC (exception from informed
    consent) research, 37–42
Eli Lilly, 130

emergency settings: research in, 37–42
Emanuel, Ezekiel, 29
Environmental Protection Agency: lead
    paint studies, 119–123
epistemic injustice, 192–193
Epstein, Steven, 190
equal treatment, 3–4
equity, 91–92
Ethical Principles and Guidelines for the
    Protection of Human Subjects
    of Research (Belmont Report)
    (National Commission), 1–2, 7,
    17–18, 25, 28, 78–79, 125–127,
    157, 170–171, 188–189, 202
ethical review committees, 182–183
ethical principles, 157, 173
    cultural differences in, 101, 182–183
    double standards, 9, 173
    international guidelines, 177–180, 184
    public perspectives on, 61–63
    training in, 171
ethnic minorities, 211. See also race
    and racism
    Policy and Guidelines on the
        Inclusion of Women and
        Minorities as Subjects in Clinical
        Research, 27–28
    requirements for inclusion of, 26–27
evaluation of research, 213
exception from informed consent
    (EFIC), 37–42
Experimentation with Human
    Beings: The Authority of the
    Investigator, Subject, Profession,
    and State in the Human
    Experimentation Process (Katz,
    Capron, and Glass), 15–16
exploitation, 189

Faden, Ruth, 195–197, 202
fair benefits framework, 176–177,
    180–182

fairness, 184
  in distribution of risks and benefits,
      2–4, 13–14, 93, 125–126
    for children, 72–73
    historical examination of, 16–20
    after study completion, 18–20
  in selection of subjects, 2, 13–14, 16–20
family surrogates, 61–63
Farfel, Mark, 120
Fast Track program, 43
FDA. *See* Federal Drug Administration;
      Food and Drug Administration
FDCA (Federal Food, Drug, and
      Cosmetic Act), 77, 83
federal advisory committees, 28–29
Federal Drug Administration (FDA), 27
Federal Food, Drug, and Cosmetic Act
      (FDCA), 77, 83
Federalwide Assurance (FWA), 26
Fee, Elizabeth, 117–118
feminism, 190
Walter E. Fernald State School (Boston,
      MA), 6, 75–76, 82
fetal
  protections, 6–7, 18, 26–27
  safety, 97–98
Fett, Sharla, 116
financial resources, 193, 210, 214
financial settlements, 140, 156, 163–164
Finland, 174–175
First Nations populations, 138
Fogarty International Center, 171
follow-up: post-trial responsibilities,
      9, 18–20
Food and Drug Administration (FDA),
      38, 76–78, 79n, 84, 161–162
  Accelerated Approval program, 43
  drug approval process, 124–125
  Fast Track program, 43
  FDA Modernization Act (FDAMA), 83, 93
  FDA Reauthorization Act, 83–84

FDA Safety and Innovation Act, 83–84
  guidelines for industry on pregnant
      women in clinical trials, 101
  guidelines for new drug
      applications, 99–100
  Pediatric Rule, 83–84
  policies regarding inclusion of
      women, 99, 101
  Priority Review program, 43
  requirements for pediatric
      labeling, 83
  strategies to improve recruitment
      of women and minorities into
      clinical trials, 100
  Treatment Investigational New Drug
      (Treatment IND) program, 43
Food and Drugs Act, 77
Ford Foundation, 211
Fort Detrick, 160–161
France, 175–176
Fricker, Miranda, 192–193
funding, 193, 210, 214
future directions
  for African American participation in
      research, 125–131
  for community engagement, 145–147
  for global research, 183–184
  for military research, 165
  for pediatric research, 85–86
  for research in acute, emergent
      illnesses, 40–42
  for research in patients with poor
      prognoses, 44–45
  for research in Phase I trials with sick
      patients, 48–49
  for research in populations with
      cognitive impairment, 63–66
  for research with convenient and
      captive populations, 165–166
  for women's participation, 103
FWA. *See* Federalwide Assurance

Gartler, Stanley, 118
gender justice, 101
gender representation, 211
Genetic Information Non-
    Discrimination Act, 136
genetic research, 135–136, 138
genomic data sharing, 20, 119
Gey, George, 116
Ghana, 145
Glasgow, Scotland, 198
Glass, Eleanor Swift, 15–16
global health, 198–200
global research, 169–186
Good Participatory Practice Guidelines
    (GPP), 137–138
Government Accountability Office
    (GAO), 27
Government Accounting Office (GAO), 27
government-sponsored research, 211
GPP (Good Participatory Practice
    Guidelines), 137–138
Grassley, Charles, 39
Greenwald, Anthony, 124
Grimes v. Kennedy Krieger Institute, Inc.,
    7, 119–123, 129
Guatemala: Sexually Transmitted
    Disease Inoculation Study, 8–9,
    23–24, 164–165
guidelines for research, international,
    177–180, 184
"Guidelines for the Ethical Conduct
    of Studies to Evaluate Drugs
    in Pediatric Populations"
    (AAP), 82–83
Gulf War Syndrome, 161–162

Hansen disease, 8–9
Harkness, Jon, 157
Havasupai tribe, 140
health care, 123–124
health, global, 198–200

health research, 187–207. *See also*
    research
    allocation of resources to, 193
    global, 169–186
    spending gap, 200
    theories of justice in, 193–203
Health Services Research
    Administration, 22
HeLa cells, 7, 115–119, 130
HeLa Genome Data Access Working
    Group, 119
Heller, Jean, 113
hemorrhagic shock research, 38–39
Hendrix, Thomas, 122–123
hepatitis studies: at Willowbrook State
    School (Staten Island, NY), 3, 6,
    16, 74–75, 82
historical perspectives
    on community engagement,
        136–145
    on global research, 170–183
    on justice in research, 8–9, 14–29
    on pediatric research, 74–76
    on pharmaceutical
        regulation, 76–78
    on prison experiments, 154–158
    on racism, 113–123
    on research in populations with
        cognitive impairment, 55–57
    on research with vulnerable
        sick, 37–39
    on women's participation, 92–98
HIV Prevention Trials Network
    (HPTN), 180
HIV/AIDS activism, 8
HIV/AIDS advocacy, 190
HIV/AIDS research
    azidothymidine (AZT) studies,
        172–173
    community engagement in, 137–138,
        145–146

HIV/AIDS research (*Cont.*)
  future directions, 44–45, 145–146
  Good Participatory Practice
      Guidelines (GPP), 137–138
  historical examination of, 42–44, 95–96
  prevention research, 136, 179–180
  requirements for Community
      Advisory Boards (CABs), 137
  women's participation in, 95–96
hospitalized patients: research with, 152
HPTN (HIV Prevention Trials
      Network), 180
human subjects, 213. *See also specific*
      populations; specific studies
  compensatory justice towards, 14
  convenient and captive populations,
      152–168
  decisionally impaired adults, 54–55
  distribution of risks and benefits to, 2–4,
      13–14, 16–20, 72–73, 93, 125–126
  distributive justice-based arguments
      for right to participate in
      research, 189–190
  Experimentation with Human
      Beings: The Authority of the
      Investigator, Subject, Profession,
      and State in the Human
      Experimentation Process (Katz,
      Capron, and Glass), 15–16
  guidelines on pregnant women in
      clinical trials, 101
  Guidance Point 15, 19, 179–180
  history of research with, 14–29
  mentally disabled persons, 55
  Policy and Guidelines on the Inclusion
      of Children as Participants in
      Research Involving Human
      Subjects, 27–28
  Policy and Guidelines on the
      Inclusion of Women and
      Minorities as Subjects in Clinical
      Research, 27–28

  post-trial benefits, 18–20, 176–182
  recruitment of, 211, 214
  regulations on protection of,
      78–82, 214
  research with, 5
  respect for, 140–141
  retention of, 214
  selection of, 2, 16–20
    distributive justice in, 188–189
    fair, 13–14
  sick patients
    with acute, emergent
        illnesses, 37–42
    Phase I trials with, 45–49
    with poor prognoses, 42–45
  strategies to improve recruitment
      of women and minorities into
      clinical trials, 100
  vulnerable subjects, 24, 26–28, 36–53
  women, 6–7, 91–111, 115–119
humanitarian assistance, 200

ideal theory, 201
incapacity, 64
India, 169–170
Indian Health Services, 138
individual justice, 2
industrialized nations, 169–170, 172–176
industry-sponsored research, 171, 210
infectious hepatitis studies: at
      Willowbrook State School (Staten
      Island, NY), 3, 6, 16, 74–75, 82
informed consent
  in combat conditions, 161
  exception from informed consent
      (EFIC), 37–42
  waivers, 161
informed volunteers, 158
injury: remedies for, 20–22
injustice, 2
  epistemic, 192–193
  unjust disadvantage, 197

Institute of Medicine (IOM), 27, 80, 95
  recommendations for prison
    research, 158
  *Unequal Treatment: Confronting Racial
    and Ethnic Disparities in Health
    Care*, 123
institutional approaches, 138–139
institutional review boards (IRBs), 38,
    120, 122–123, 182–183, 208, 211
  criteria for approval of research, 17–18
  establishment of, 25
  future directions for, 129
  historical examination of, 24–26
  recommendations for, 29
  requirements for, 25–26, 79–80, 158
institutionalized subjects. *See also*
    convenient and captive populations
  children, 74
  research with, 8–9, 152–168
    current context, 59
    historical reviews, 56, 74–76
international guidelines, 177–180, 184
Inuit populations, 138
Investigational New Drugs (INDs), 43
IRBs. *See* institutional review boards
Ivy, Andrew, 155

Japan, 198
Jewish Chronic Disease Hospital
    (Brooklyn, NY), 3, 15
Jews and Jewish community, 135–136
Johns Hopkins Hospital, 116–117
Johns Hopkins University, 120
Joint United Nations Programme on
    HIV/AIDS (UNAIDS), 137–138
Jones, James, 15, 114, 117
Journal of Legal Medicine, 155
journals, 212
justice
  and community research, 135–151
  compensatory, 3, 14, 20–24, 92
  debates over, 188–193

definition of, 4
distributive, 7–8, 13–14, 17, 208
  arguments for right to participate
    in research, 189–190
  in global research, 170
  historical examination of, 16–20
  in subject selection, 188–189
  and women's participation, 91–92
  as fairness in distribution, 125–126
gender, 101
in global research, 169–186
in health research, 187–207
individual, 2
  obligations of, 199
in pediatric research, 72–90
principles of, 2–3, 188–193
procedural, 14, 24–29, 182–183
and race and racism, 112–134
as reciprocity, 19
in research
  evolution of, 13–35
  examination of, 1–12
  implementation of, 209–212
  pursuit of, 208–215
  suggestions for implementation of,
    212–213
in research with convenient and
    captive populations, 152–168
in research with populations with
    cognitive impairment, 54–71
in research with vulnerable sick, 36–53
restorative, 23
theories of, 193–203
and women's participation, 91–111

Kahn, Jonathan, 124–125
Kass, Nancy, 6–7
Katz, Jay, 15–16
Kennedy, Edward (Ted), 16–17
Kennedy Krieger Institute (KKI): lead
    paint study, 7, 119–123, 129
Kim, Scott, 5

King, Katherine, 8
King, Patricia, 7, 18
Krugman, Saul, 16, 74–75

Lacks, Deborah, 116, 130
Lacks, Henrietta, 7, 115–119
Landecker, Hannah, 117
LAR (legally authorized representative), 55, 59–62
Lasagna, Louis, 44, 156
Lasagna Report (National Committee to Review Current Procedures for Approval of New Drugs for Cancer and AIDS), 43–44
Lavery, James, 8
lead paint study (Kennedy Krieger Institute), 7, 119–123, 129
lead poisoning, 120
Lead Wars: The Politics of Science and the Fate of America's Children (Markowitz and Rosner), 120–123
leadership, 102, 104
learning healthcare systems (LHS), 202–203
legal issues, 101–102
legally authorized representative (LAR), 55, 59–62
legislation, 84–86
legitimacy, 142, 147
Levine, Robert J., 135, 157
LHS (learning healthcare systems), 202–203
liability concerns, 101–102
life expectancy, 198
Little, Margaret Olivia, 101
low and middle-income countries (LMIC), 169–170
industry-sponsored research in, 171
risk-benefit ratios, 172–176
low-resource countries, 169–170
LSD (lysergic acid diethylamide) studies, 121, 160

Lyerly, Anne Drapkin, 6–7
lysergic acid diethylamide (LSD) studies, 121, 160

Macklin, Ruth, 9
malaria research
prison experiments, 154
women's participation in, 97
male bias, 93–94, 101
Markowitz, Gerald, 120–123
Marmot, Michael, 192
Marston, Robert Q., 25
Martucci, Jessica, 192
Maryland, 57
Massachusetts Task Force on Human Subjects Research, 75–76
Matsuda, Mari, 130
maximum tolerated dose (MTD), 45–46
McCarthy, Charles, 3
M.D. Anderson Hospital, 46
medical leadership, 102
mentally disabled persons: research with
current context, 57–59
future directions, 66
historical review, 55–57
at Willowbrook State School (Staten Island, NY), 3, 6, 16, 74–75, 82
Meslin, Eric, 3
Métis populations, 138
Mexico, 145
military personnel: research with, 121, 152, 158–162, 165
military research, 165
Miller, Frank, 194
minimal risk, 79–81
minorities, 211. *See also* race and racism
Policy and Guidelines on the Inclusion of Women and Minorities as Subjects in Clinical Research, 27–28
requirements for inclusion of, 26–27

Mississippi: prison experiments, 154
morality, 139–143
Moreno, Jonathan, 8–9
morning sickness, 97
multidrug-resistant tuberculosis research, 157
mushroom-cloud–penetration experiments, 160

Nagel, Thomas, 199
National Academy of Medicine, 27, 80, 95. *See also* Institute of Medicine (IOM)
National Academy of Sciences, Engineering, and Medicine, 27
National Bioethics Advisory Commission (NBAC), 19, 21–22, 29, 57, 61, 138
National Bioethics Center, 130
National Center for Bioethics in Research and Health Care, 23
National Commission for the Protection of Human Subjects of Biomedical and Behavioral Research, 1–4, 28, 56, 78–82, 125–126, 135
    Belmont Report (Ethical Principles and Guidelines for the Protection of Human Subjects of Research), 1–2, 7, 17–18, 25, 28, 78–79, 125–127, 157, 170–171, 188–189, 202
    definition of minimal risk, 79–80
    recommendations against prison experiments, 156
    Research Involving Children, 79
National Committee to Review Current Procedures for Approval of New Drugs for Cancer and AIDS, 43–44
National Human Research Protections Advisory Committee, 80
National Institute of Allergy and Infectious Disease (NIAID), 137

National Institute on Aging, 60
National Institutes of Health (NIH), 25, 27, 45, 119, 171, 210
    azidothymidine (AZT) studies, 172–173
    Clinical and Translational Science Awards (CTSAs), 102
    Clinical Center, 16, 171
    Final Genomic Data Sharing Policy, 20
    guidelines addressing gender in research, 98
    leadership, 102
    Office of Research on Women's Health (ORWH), 98–99, 103
    off-patent program, 83
    Policy and Guidelines on the Inclusion of Children as Participants in Research Involving Human Subjects, 27–28
    Policy and Guidelines on the Inclusion of Women and Minorities as Subjects in Clinical Research, 27–28
    policy guidelines, 83–85
    requirements for CABs, 137
    requirements for community engagement, 138–139
    Yellow Book, DHEW, 25
National Institutes of Health Revitalization Act, 26–27
National Research Act, 3, 16–17, 56, 78
National Vaccine Injury Compensation Program, 22
Navajo miners and millers: research with, 121, 152
Navrongo Health Research Centre, 145
Nazi Germany, 154–155
NBAC (National Bioethics Advisory Commission), 19, 21–22, 29, 138
Nelson, Robert, 6
neonates, 18
Nevada, 160

*New England Journal of Medicine
(NEJM)*, 14–15
New Jersey, 57, 61
New York State, 57, 156
New York Times, 15, 42
Newman, Peter, 145–146
The Nicomachean Ethics (Aristotle), 4
NIH. *See* National Institutes of Health
NIH Revitalization Act, 99, 126
nonideal theories, 201
nonoppression and nondomination,
190–193
Northfield Labs, 38
Nuffield Council on Bioethics, 19–20
Nuremberg Code, 155, 159–160
Nuremberg War Crimes Trials, 14, 154

Obama, Barack, 24, 55, 128, 164–165
observational studies, 154
Obstetrics and Gynecology, 102
Office for Protection from Research
Risks (OPRR), 26
Office of Human Research Protections
(OHRP), 26, 60
Office of Management and Budget
(OMB), 126
Office of Research on Women's Health
(ORWH), 98–99, 103
Office of the Surgeon General, 161
OHRP (Office of Human Research
Protections), 26, 60
older persons, 103
O'Leary, Hazel, 23
oncology research, 5, 46–49
Operation Desert Shield, 161
Operation Desert Storm, 161–162
oppression, 127–128
principles of nonoppression and
nondomination, 190–193
of women, 92
OPRR (Office for Protection from
Research Risks), 26

Oregon: prison experiments, 155
ORWH (Office of Research on
Women's Health), 98–99, 103
ovarian cancer studies, 135–136
overprotection, 7–8

Pan American Sanitary Bureau (now
the Pan American Health
Organization): Sexually
Transmitted Disease Inoculation
Study (Guatemala studies), 8–9,
23–24, 164–165
participants. *See* risk-benefit ratios
participatory research, 143–144
paternalism, 190
patient-led research (PLR), 192–194
pediatric labeling, 72–73, 83
pediatric research, 6–7, 72–90
acceptable levels of risks and
potential benefits, 61
current trends, 84–85
evaluation of fairness in, 72–73
future directions, 85–86
Guatemala Sexually Transmitted
Disease Inoculation Study, 8–9,
23–24, 164–165
guidelines for, 83–85
"Guidelines for the Ethical Conduct
of Studies to Evaluate Drugs
in Pediatric Populations"
(AAP), 82–83
historical perspectives on, 55–56, 74–76
Kennedy Krieger Institute lead paint
study, 7, 119–123
Policy and Guidelines on the Inclusion
of Children as Participants in
Research Involving Human
Subjects, 27–28
regulatory protections for, 18
requirements for, 26–28, 79–80
Research Involving Children (National
Commission), 79

Willowbrook State School, 74–75
at Walter E. Fernald State School, 6,
    75–76, 82
at Willowbrook State School, 3, 6, 16,
    74–75, 82
Pediatric Research Equity Act
    (PREA), 83–84
Pediatric Rule, 83–84
peer review, 212
pellagra studies, 154
Pettit, Philip, 191
Pharmaceutical Manufacturers
    Association, 155
pharmaceutical regulation, 76–78
Phase I trials, 5, 45–46
    consent-related challenges, 46–47
    prison experiments, 155
    with sick patients, 45–49
Phase II trials, 45–46, 99
Phase III trials, 99
Phase IV trials, 97
Philippines: prison experiments, 154
PHS Policy and Procedure Order #
    129, 16
Physicians' Desk Reference, 73, 83
placebos, 173–174
PLR (patient-led research), 192–194
policy, 13–14
    Basic Policy, 25
    future directions, 103
    on women's participation,
        27–28, 98–100
Policy and Guidelines on the Inclusion
    of Children as Participants in
    Research Involving Human
    Subjects, 27
Policy and Guidelines on the Inclusion
    of Women and Minorities
    as Subjects in Clinical
    Research, 27–28
political correctness, 182
political movements, 13

Pollak, Joanne, 120
PolyHeme®, 38–39
Powers, Madison, 195–197
Pratt, Bridget, 196
PREA (Pediatric Research Equity
    Act), 83–84
Precision Medicine Initiative (All of Us
    Research Program), 128
pregnancy research, 96–98, 101
pregnant women
    federal policies specific to, 100–101
    regulatory protections applying to, 18
    as vulnerable subjects, 26–27
prejudice, 192–193. See also race
    and racism
President's Advisory Committee
    on Human Radiation
    Experiments, 155
President's Commission for the Study
    of Bioethical Issues (PCSBI),
    21–22, 24, 55, 138, 164–165
President's Commission for the Study
    of Ethical Problems in Medicine
    and Biomedical and Behavioral
    Research, 21–22, 28, 56
Principal Investigators, 102
prioritization, 193, 210–211
Priority Review program, 43
prison research, 8–9, 18, 24, 26, 55, 78, 82,
    91, 126, 152-158, 164–166, 188–189
    future directions, 165
    history of, 154–158
    protections related to prisoners, 18
    requirements for, 156–157
private sector funding, 210
procedural justice, 14, 24–29, 182–183
program evaluation, 165
Protecting Human Subjects (President's
    Commission for the Study of
    Ethical Problems in Medicine
    and Biomedical and Behavioral
    Research), 28

protectionism, 3, 9
  towards convenient and captive
    populations, 166
  evolution of, 214
  fetal protection, 6–7
  US research regulations on human
    subject protection, 78–82
  towards vulnerable subjects, 26–28
  towards women, 92
proxy directives, 65–66
Public Access Defibrillation Trial, 38
public perspectives, 61–63
pyridostigmine bromide (PB), 161

quality assessment, 165
questions, scientific, 213

race and racism, 7, 102–103, 112–134
  Policy and Guidelines on the
    Inclusion of Women and
    Minorities as Subjects in Clinical
    Research, 27–28
  requirements for inclusion of racial
    minorities, 26–27
  Unequal Treatment: Confronting Racial
    and Ethnic Disparities in Health
    Care (IOM), 123–124
radiation experiments
  Advisory Committee on Human
    Radiation Experiments
    (ACHRE), 21–22, 75–76
  apology for, 22–23
  with Navajo miners and millers,
    121, 152
  prison experiments, 155
  recommendations for, 22
  at Walter E. Fernald State School, 6,
    75–76, 82
Ramsey, Paul, 75
randomized controlled trials (RCTs), 43
rape victims, 182–183

Rawls, John, 195–196, 201
reciprocity, 19
recruitment of subjects, 100, 211, 214
Reed, Walter, 159
regulations
  Code of Federal Regulations, 79n
  definition of minimal risk, 79–80
  EFIC (exception from informed
    consent), 37–39
  for federal research, 18–19
  pharmaceutical, 76–78
  for protection of research subjects,
    78–82, 214
  for research review, 165–166
remedies for injury, 20–22
representation, 40
research
  with aboriginal populations, 138
  acceptable risks and benefits, 61–63
  in acute, emergent illnesses, 37–42
  African American participation in,
    123–131
  allocation of risks and burdens in, 202
  community engagement, 8, 135–151
  with convenient and captive
    populations, 8–9, 152–168
  in emergency settings, 37, 40–42
  equity in, 91–92
  evaluation of, 213
  experiments of opportunity, 154
  future directions, 40–42
  gender representation in, 211
  global, 169–186
  government-sponsored, 211
  health, 187–207
  with human subjects, 5, 14–29
  industry-sponsored, 171, 210
  international ethical guidelines for,
    177–180, 184
  justice in
    evolution of, 13–35

examination of, 1–12
implementation of, 209–212
pursuit of, 208–215
suggestions for implementation of,
212–213
theories about, 169–186
minority representation in, 211
participation in, 211, 213
distributive justice-based
arguments for right of,
189–190
fair distribution of risks and
benefits in, 2–4, 13–14, 16–20,
72–73, 93, 125–126
obligations for, 202–203
participatory, 143–144
patient-led (PLR), 192–194
pediatric, 72–90
in populations with cognitive
impairment, 54–71
post-trial benefits, 18–20, 176–182
post-trial responsibilities, 9, 18–20
priorities for, 193, 210–211
race and racism in, 112–134
regulations on (*see* regulations)
risk-benefit profiles, 61
selection of subjects for, 2
social contracts for, 194
spending gap, 200
subjects of (*see* human subjects)
training in ethics for, 171
with vulnerable sick, 36–53
in women's health issues, 26–27
women's participation in, 91–111
research communities, 143
Research Involving Children (National
Commission), 79
*Research Involving Persons with
Mental Disorders that May
Affect Decisionmaking Capacity*
(NBAC), 29

research proxy, 65
research review. *See* review
resource-poor countries, 169–170
resources: allocation of, 193, 214
respect, 140–141
restorative justice, 23
retention issues, 214
Reverby, Susan, 24, 131, 164–165
review
ethical review committees, 182–183
by institutional review boards (IRBs),
211 (*see also* institutional review
boards (IRBs))
peer review, 212
regulations for, 165–166
Rhodes, Rosamond, 201–202
rights
to participate in research, 189–190
universal, 200
risk-benefit ratios, 172–176
acceptable risks and benefits,
40–41, 61–63
allocation of risks and burdens, 202
fair benefits framework, 176–177,
180–182
fair distribution, 2–4, 13–14, 16–20,
72–73, 93, 125–126
historical examination of, 16–20
minimal risk, 79–81
nonobvious risks and benefits,
139–140
post-trial benefits, 18–20, 176–182
and pregnancy, 101
public perspectives, 61–63
unresolved issues, 61–62
Rivera, Geraldo, 16
Rosner, David, 120–123
Ross, Lainie Friedman, 6
rotavirus vaccine, 174–175
Rothman, David, 75
RU-486 trials, 175–176

SACHRP (Secretary's Advisory
    Committee on Human Research
    Protections), 61, 80
safety
  FDA Safety and Innovation Act, 83–84
  fetal, 97–98
Saghai, Yashar, 9–10
scarlet fever research, 154
science, 192
scientific leadership, 102
scientific questions, 213
Secretary's Advisory Committee on
    Human Research Protections
    (SACHRP), 80
sex differences, 92–94
sex workers
  Guatemala Sexually Transmitted
    Disease Inoculation Study, 8–9,
    23–24, 164–165
  tenofovir PrEP trials with, 136, 140–141
sexually transmitted infections (STIs)
  Guatemala Sexually Transmitted
    Disease Inoculation Study, 8–9,
    23–24, 164–165
  prison experiments, 154
  Tuskegee Syphilis Study (Study of
    Untreated Syphilis in the Negro
    Male), 3, 7, 15, 23, 78, 113–115,
    121, 125, 130–131, 152
Shannon, James, 16, 24–25
sharing data, 20
shock, hemorrhagic: PolyHeme®
    trials, 38–39
Sibelius, Kathleen, 23–24, 164–165
Sierra Leone, 198
Skloot, Rebecca, 116–117
social contracts, 194, 201
social forces, 103
social values, 192
soldiers: research with, 121, 152–153,
    158–162, 165
Southam, Chester, 15

spending gap, 200
standards
  double, 9, 173
  ethical, 173
statism, 199
Stewart, William, 16
STIs. See sexually transmitted
    infections
students: research with, 152, 162–165
subjects of research. See human
    subjects
sub-Saharan Africa, 169–170
surrogates
  of consent, 61–63
  de facto, 65
syphilis, 117
  Tuskegee Syphilis Study (Study of
    Untreated Syphilis in the Negro
    Male), 3, 7, 15, 23, 78, 113–115,
    121, 125, 130–131, 152

T. D. v. New York Department of Mental
    Health, 57
Task Force of Public Health Service
    Employees, 25
Task Force on Research Specific to
    Pregnant and Lactating Women
    (PRGLAC), 100
10/90 gap, 200
tenofovir research, 136, 140–141
thalidomide, 6–7, 101–102
The Immortal Life of Henrietta Lacks
    (Skloot), 116–117
theories of justice, 193–203
therapeutic research, 60. See also
    research
training and training programs, 171
Treatment Investigational New Drug
    (Treatment IND) program, 43
trends, 84–85
trust, 7–8
tuberculosis research, 157

Turtle, Robert, 81
Tuskegee Syphilis Study (Study of
    Untreated Syphilis in the Negro
    Male), 3, 7, 15, 78, 113–115, 121,
    130–131, 152
  apology for, 23
  response to, 125
Tuskegee Syphilis Study Ad Hoc
    Advisory Panel, 15–17, 21, 115
Tuskegee University, 23, 130
typhus and typhoid research, 154

UNAIDS (Joint United Nations
    Programme on HIV/ AIDS),
    137–138, 179–180
unconscious subjects, 55–56
*Unequal Treatment: Confronting Racial
    and Ethnic Disparities in Health
    Care* (IOM), 123
United Kingdom, 19–20
United States
  government-sponsored research, 211
  prison experiments, 155–156
  research policy, 13–14
  research regulations, 13, 17–19, 26,
    56, 78, 189
  research review regulations, 165–166
  research with military personnel, 159
United States Air Force, 160
United States Army, 121, 160–161
United States Public Health Service
    (USPHS)
  PHS Policy and Procedure Order # 129, 16
  Sexually Transmitted Disease
    Inoculation Study (Guatemala
    study), 8–9, 23–24, 164–165
  Tuskegee Syphilis Study (Study of
    Untreated Syphilis in the Negro
    Male), 3, 7, 15, 23, 78, 113–115,
    121, 125, 130–131, 152
United States Supreme Court, 160
universal rights, 200

University of California at San
    Francisco, 136
University of California, Los Angeles
    (UCLA), 57
unjust disadvantage, 197
unresolved issues
  regarding LARs, 61–62
  regarding risk-benefit
    considerations, 61–62
  research in populations with
    cognitive impairment, 59–61
uranium experiments, 121, 152

vaccines
  AIDS Vaccine Advocacy Coalition
    (AVAC), 137–138
  National Vaccine Injury
    Compensation Program, 22
  rotavirus, 174–175
values, 192, 213
Venereal Disease Research Laboratory
    (VDRL): Sexually Transmitted
    Disease Inoculation Study
    (Guatemala studies), 8–9, 23–24,
    164–165
venereal diseases, 117–118
Virginia, 57, 61
volunteer subjects
  military personnel, 158–160
  prison inmates, 156
vulnerability, 81–82, 190
vulnerable subjects or
    populations, 2, 7–8
  aboriginal populations, 138
  children, 6–7, 61, 72–90
  convenient and captive populations,
    152–168
  decisionally impaired adults, 54–55
  mentally disabled persons, 55
  older persons, 103
  populations with cognitive
    impairment, 54–71

vulnerable subjects or
populations (*Cont.*)
requirements for inclusion of,
24, 26–28
research with, 36–53
sick patients: Phase I trials with, 45–49
sick patients with acute, emergent
illnesses, 37–42
sick patients with poor
prognoses, 42–45
subgroups of women, 102–103

Washington State: prison
experiments, 155
wealthy countries, 169–170
well-being: core elements necessary for, 197
Whistleblowing in Biomedical Research
(President's Commission for
the Study of Ethical Problems in
Medicine and Biomedical and
Behavioral Research), 28
Willowbrook State School (Staten
Island, NY), 3, 6, 16, 74–75, 82
women
Henrietta Lacks, 115–119
oppression of, 92, 101, 182, 191–192
pregnant
federal policies specific to, 100–101
regulatory protections
applying to, 18
as vulnerable subjects, 26–27
rape victims, 182–183
sex workers
Guatemala Sexually Transmitted
Disease Inoculation Study, 8–9,
23–24, 164–165

tenofovir PrEP trials with, 136,
140–141
women's health issues, 92–93, 101
cardiovascular disease, 94–95
HIV disease, 95–96
limitations on research on, 26–27
Office of Research on Women's
Health (ORWH), 98–99, 103
pregnancy, 96–98, 101
RU-486 trials, 175–176
women's participation, 6–7, 91–111,
191–192
cultural factors, 101
federal research policy on, 98–100
future directions for, 103–104
guidelines for, 98
historical examination of, 92–98
in leadership, 102
liability concerns, 101–102
Policy and Guidelines on the
Inclusion of Women and
Minorities as Subjects in Clinical
Research, 27–28
requirements for, 26–27
in research, 102
World Health Organization (WHO)
Guidance Point 19, 179–180
RU-486 analog trials, 176
training in research ethics, 171
World Medical Association
(WMA): Declaration of Helsinki
(DoH), 20, 155, 172, 177–178

Yellow Book (NIH), 24–25
yellow fever research, 159
Young, Iris Marion, 92, 127, 190